Clinical

Clinical Haematology:
a Postgraduate Exam Companion

Drew Provan MB MRCP (UK) MRCPath

Consultant Haematologist, Honorary Senior Lecturer
Southampton University Hospitals NHS Trust, UK

Andrew Amos MB MRCP (UK) DTM&H

Senior Registrar in Haematology
Southampton University Hospitals NHS Trust, UK

Alastair Smith BSc (Hons) MB FRCP (Glas & Lond) FRCPath

Consultant Haematologist, Honorary Senior Lecturer
Southampton University Hospitals NHS Trust, UK

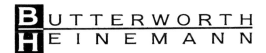

Butterworth-Heinemann
Linacre House, Jordan Hill, Oxford OX2 8DP
A division of Reed Educational and Professional Publishing Ltd

Ɋ A member of the Reed Elsevier plc group

OXFORD   BOSTON   JOHANNESBURG
MELBOURNE   NEW DELHI   SINGAPORE

First published 1997

British Library Cataloguing in Publication Data
A catalogue record for this book is available from the British Library

ISBN 0 7506 2920 7

Library of Congress Cataloguing in Publication Data
A catalogue record for this book is available from the Library of Congress

Typeset by David Gregson Associates, Beccles, Suffolk
Printed and bound in Great Britain by The University Press, Cambridge

Contents

Preface

In common with most medical specialties, clinical haematology relies on pattern recognition. The material encountered in the clinic and on the wards typically involves clinical history and physical examination as well as haematological, biochemical and immunological data. By piecing these together the haematologist formulates a working diagnosis. So, too, in this book we have provided clinical scenarios accompanied by relevant investigation data to enable examination candidates to generate a clinical diagnosis which, we hope, will improve examination skills for both the MRCP and MRCPath examinations.

We recognize that the requirements for the MRCP and MRCPath candidate differ and for this reason we have attempted to customize the explanations with both types of examination candidate in mind. In order to achieve this we have provided 'small-print' detail set in smaller type for the MRCPath candidate, which may be ignored by those studying for the MRCP examination since the MRCPath candidate requires detailed knowledge of haematological, immunophenotypic and karyotypic features associated with haematological disease. There are a few questions that are specifically intended for MRCPath; these include blood transfusion questions and those questions in which immuno-phenotypic data are presented.

The clinical cases are written very much in the style of the MRCP written examination and we have used a layout which we feel closely mimics that examination. The explanations, we hope, are sufficiently detailed to provide background information relating to the disorder being discussed. However, this is not a textbook and candidates should refer to larger texts if further information is required. These are listed towards the end of the book.

We have included an Examination Lists section (Chapter 8) which provides lists useful for written and other examinations. In the Review articles (Chapter 7) we have provided synopses of specific areas which we hope will be useful for written and oral examinations.

We welcome comments or suggestions for future revisions of this book. If there are errors in the text then we bear full responsibility and would, again, welcome constructive criticism if mistakes are detected.

DP
TAA
AGS

Acknowledgements

We are indebted to many of our colleagues for providing clinical data and material for this book. In particular we would like to thank Dr Ben Mead, Department of Medical Oncology, Royal South Hants Hospital and Dr Frank Boulton, Director of Wessex BTS for providing cases and Dr Liz Hodges for immunophenotypic profiles. Dr Rebecca Frewin and Dr Rania Katapodis, our overworked Registrar and SHO, helped with slide, data and clinical case sections. Dr Sue O'Connell, Department of Virology, Southampton General Hospital, provided assistance with questions relating to viral serology. We are grateful to Dr Fiona Ross, Wessex Regional Cytogenetics, Salisbury District Hospital, Salisbury for providing karyotypic data. Dr Odurny, Consultant Radiologist at Southampton General Hospital, kindly provided us with some of the radiological material. Dr Dina Choudhury contributed slide material. We are grateful to Organon Teknika for kind permission to photograph the Simplate bleeding time device.

We are grateful to Mrs Shirley Mirakian for secretarial support and to Mr Tim Brown of Butterworth-Heinemann for taking on this project in the first place.

Note

Slide questions 4, 12, 16 and 18 and data interpretation questions 11, 16, 19, 33, 38, 39 and 40 are intended for the MRCPath rather than MRCP candidate. The MRCP candidate should feel free to try the questions but can be assured that detailed blood transfusion or immunophenotypic data are very unlikely to be encountered in the real MRCP examination.

Explanatory notes for MRCPath *specifically* are set in small type and can therefore safely be ignored by MRCP candidates.

Abbreviations Used

ACD	acid–citrate–dextrose
AGLT	acid glycerol lysis test
AHG	antihuman globulin
ALL	acute lymphoblastic leukaemia
AML	acute myeloid leukaemia
ANA	antinuclear antibodies
APCR	activated protein C resistance
APML	acute promyelocytic leukaemia
APTR	activated partial thromboplastin ratio
APTT	activated partial thromboplastin time
ARMS	amplification refractory mutations system
ATLL	adult T-cell leukaemia/lymphoma
ATP	adenosine triphosphate
ATRA	all-*trans* retinoic acid
B-CLL	B-cell chronic lymphocytic leukaemia
BFU-E	burst-forming unit-erythroid
BMT	bone marrow transplantation
BP	blood pressure
BUPA	British United Provident Association
cALL	common acute lymphoblastic leukaemia
CD	cluster designation
2-CDA	2-chlorodeoxyadenosine
cDNA	complementary DNA
CGL	chronic granulocytic leukaemia
CHOP	cyclophosphamide, hydroxydaunorubicin (Adriamycin), vincristine (Oncovin), prednisolone
CLL	chronic lymphocytic leukaemia
CML	chronic myeloid leukaemia
CMML	chronic myelomonocytic leukaemia
CMV	cytomegalovirus
CNS	central nervous system
CRP	C-reactive protein
CT	computerized tomography
CXR	chest radiograph
DAT	direct antiglobulin test (direct Coombs test)
dATP	deoxy ATP
DCT	direct Coombs test
DDAVP	desamino D-arginyl vasopressin
DFS	disease-free survival
DIC	disseminated intravascular coagulation
DRVVT	dilute Russell's viper venom test
DTT	dilute thromboplastin time
DVT	deep venous thrombosis
DXT	radiotherapy

EBV	Epstein–Barr Virus
ELISA	enzyme-linked immunosorbent assay
ERCP	endoscopic retrograde cholangiopancreatography
ESR	erythrocyte sedimentation rate
ET	essential thrombocythaemia
FAB	French–American–British
FACS	fluorescence-activated cell sorter
FBC	full blood count
FISH	fluorescence-*in-situ* hybridization
FITC	fluorescein-isothiocyanate
FIX	factor IX
FL	follicular lymphoma
FOB	faecal occult blood
FVIII	factor VIII
G-CSF	granulocyte-colony-stimulating factor
G6PD	glucose-6-phosphate dehydrogenase
GFR	glomerular filtration rate
GI	gastrointestinal
GM-CSF	granulocyte macrophage-colony-stimulating factor
GP	general practitioner
GPI	glycosylphosphatidylinositol
GVHD	graft-versus-host disease
Hb	haemoglobin
HbF	fetal haemoglobin
HbH	haemoglobin H (β_4)
HC2	monoclonal antibody that reacts with hairy cells
HCL	hairy cell leukaemia
HDN	haemolytic disease of the newborn
HIV	human immunodeficiency virus
HLA	human leukocyte antigen
HPA	human platelet antigen
HPFH	hereditary persistence of fetal haemoglobin
HPP	hereditary pyropoikilocytosis
HTLV-1	human T-lymphotropic virus type 1
HUS	haemolytic uraemic syndrome
IAGT	indirect antiglobulin test
IgG	immunoglobulin G
Ig JH	immunoglobulin heavy chain joining region
IL-3	interleukin-3
INR	international normalized ratio
inv	chromosomal inversion
ITP	idiopathic thrombocytopenic purpura
i.v.	intravenous
IVIg	intravenous immunoglobulin
IVU	intravenous urogram
LCR	locus control region
LDH	lactate dehydrogenase
LFTs	liver function tests

LGL	large granular lymphocyte
MAHA	microangiopathic haemolytic anaemia
McAbs	monoclonal antibodies
MCF	mean corpuscular fragility
MCH	mean corpuscular haemoglobin
MCHC	mean corpuscular haemoglobin concentration
M-CSF	macrophage colony-stimulating factor
MCV	mean cell volume
MDS	myelodysplastic syndrome
MGUS	monoclonal gammopathy of undetermined significance
MHC	major histocompatibility complex
MRI	magnetic resonance imaging
mRNA	messenger RNA
MS	multiple sclerosis
MSU	midstream urine
NADP	nicotinamide adenine diphosphate
NADPH	reduced form of NADP
NAIT	neonatal alloimmune thrombocytopenia
NHL	non-Hodgkin's lymphoma
NSAIDs	non-steroidal anti-inflammatory drugs
PA	pernicious anaemia; posteroanterior
PAS	periodic acid–Schiff
PCL	plasma cell leukaemia
PCR	polymerase chain reaction
PCV	packed cell volume
PE	phycoerythrin
PET	pre-eclamptic toxaemia
PLL	prolymphocytic leukaemia
PML	promyelocytic leukaemia
PNH	paroxysmal nocturnal haemoglobinuria
PPP	primary proliferative polycythaemia
PRV	polycythaemia rubra vera
PSA	prostate-specific antigen
PT	prothrombin time
PTP	post-transfusion purpura
RA	rheumatoid arthritis; refractory anaemia
RACE	rapid amplification of cDNA
RAEB	refractory anaemia with excess blasts
RAEB-t	refractory anaemia with excess blasts in transformation
RAR	retinoic acid receptor
RARα	retinoic acid receptor α
RARS	refractory anaemia with ring sideroblasts
RCC	red blood cell count
RXR	retinoic x receptor
rHuEPO	recombinant human erythropoietin
RiCoF	ristocetin cofactor
RSV	respiratory syncytial virus
RT-PCR	reverse transcriptase polymerase chain reaction

SCF	stem cell factor
SLE	systemic lupus erythematosus
SLVL	splenic lymphoma with villous lymphocytes
SmIg	surface membrane immunoglobulin
SVC	superior vena cava
SVCO	superior vena caval obstruction
T_4	thyroxine
TCR	T-cell receptor
TdT	terminal deoxynucleotidyl transferase
TIBC	total iron-binding capacity
TNF	tumour necrosis factor
topo II	topoisomerase II
TRAP	tartrate-resistant acid phosphatase
TSH	thyroid-stimulating hormone
TT	thrombin time
TTP	thrombotic thrombocytopenic purpura
VAD	vincristine, Adriamycin, dexamethasone
VIII:c	Factor VIII clotting activity
vWF:Ag	von Willebrand factor antigen
WBC	white blood cell count
XDPs	cross-linked fibrin degradation products

1 Slide questions

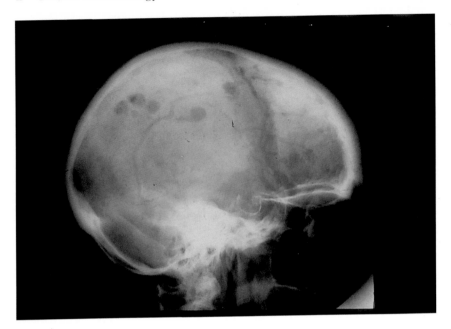

Slide 1

a. What abnormality is shown on this skull radiograph?
b. Name two disorders which may give rise to this abnormality.

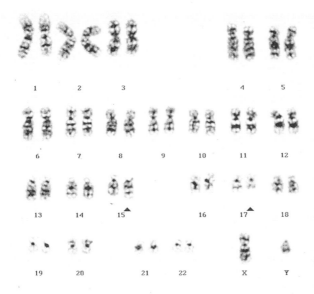

Slide 2

a. What is your interpretation of this patient's karyotype?
b. What is the likely diagnosis?
c. What is the prognosis of this condition?

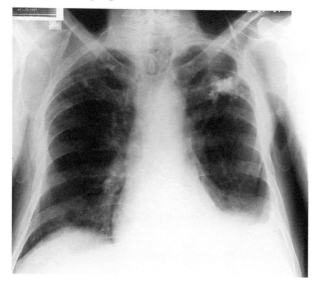

Slide 3

This patient with CLL complained of weight loss and shortness of breath.

a. Name two abnormalities on this CXR.
b. Suggest two possible causes for the radiographic appearances.

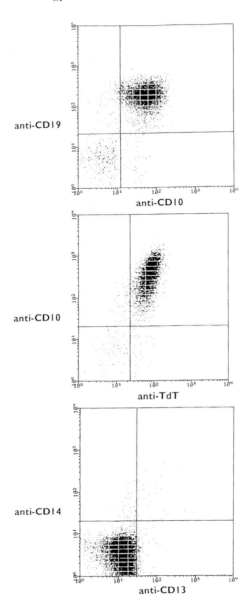

Slide 4

This is the immunophenotypic (FACS) profile from the marrow of a 4-year-old boy.

a. What is the likely underlying disorder?
b. What features would favour a good prognosis?

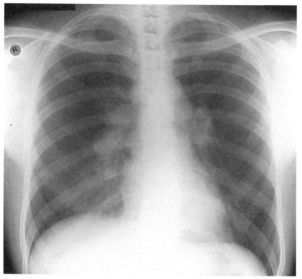

Slide 5

a. Describe the abnormality on this CXR.
b. What is your differential diagnosis?

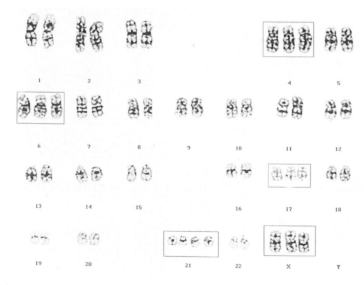

Slide 6

This is the karyotype obtained from the bone marrow of a 6-year-old girl with a haematological malignancy. Her peripheral WBC was $15 \times 10^9/l$.

a. What is the likely diagnosis?
b. What is her prognosis?

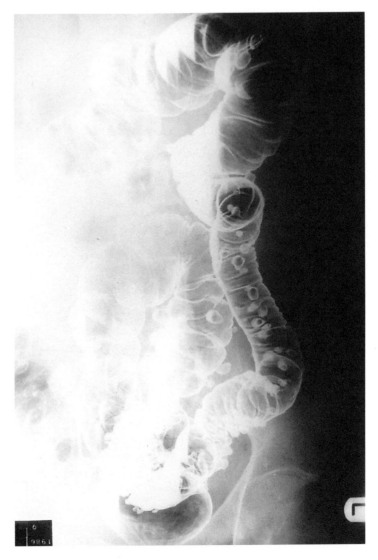

Slide 7

a. What is this investigation?
b. What abnormality is shown?
c. What are the haematological consequences of this condition?

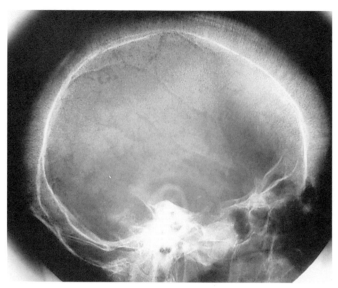

Slide 8

a. What is the major abnormality shown on this skull radiograph?
b. What is the most likely underlying condition?
c. Give two complications of this condition.

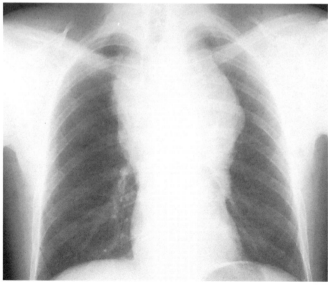

Slide 9

a. What abnormality is shown on the PA CXR?
b. Give three causes for this appearance.
c. What further investigations would you arrange?

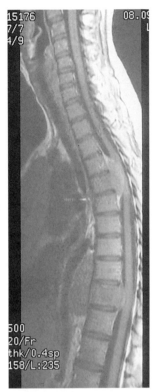

Slide 10

a. What is this investigation and what does it show?
b. Give four possible causes for this appearance.

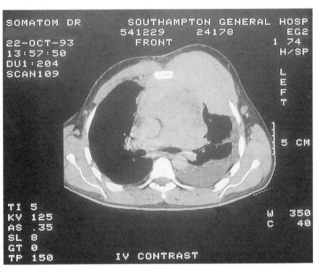

Slide 11

a. What abnormality is shown in this picture?
b. What is the likeliest cause of this appearance?

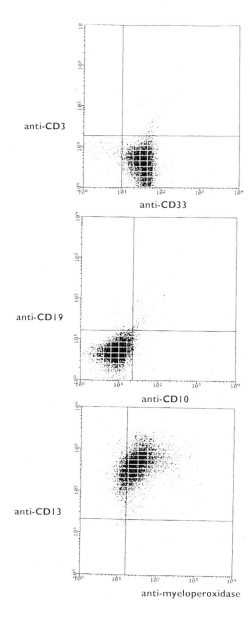

anti-CD3

anti-CD33

anti-CD19

anti-CD10

anti-CD13

anti-myeloperoxidase

Slide 12

These immunophenotypic data are from the bone marrow of a 67-year-old woman who complained of increasing tiredness.

a. What is her diagnosis?
b. Outline your initial management.

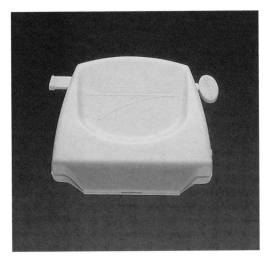

Slide 13

a. What is this device?
b. What are the indications for its use?

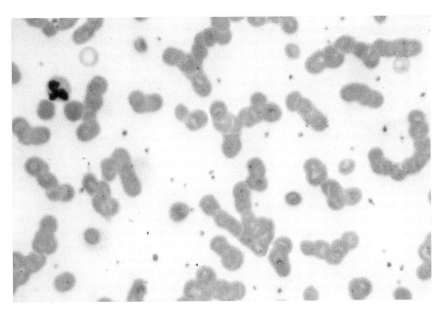

Slide 14

a. Comment on this peripheral blood film.
b. What disorders may produce this finding?
c. Suggest four investigations that would be of value.

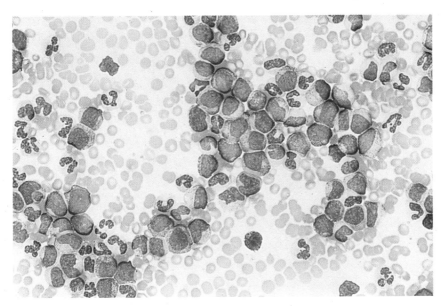

Slide 21

a. What does this peripheral blood film show?
b. What are the complications of this disorder?

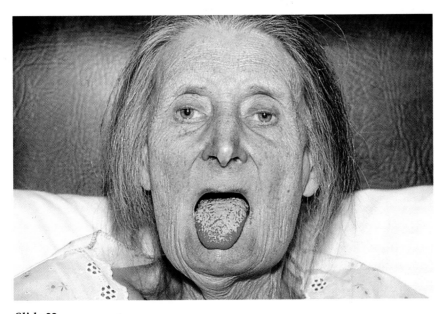

Slide 22

a. What is the principal abnormality shown in this photograph?
b. Suggest four possible causes for this appearance.

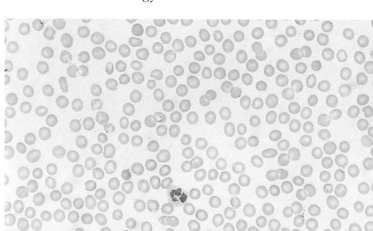

Slide 23

a. What is the most striking feature of this peripheral blood film from a 17-year-old female?
b. What condition is most likely in this age group?

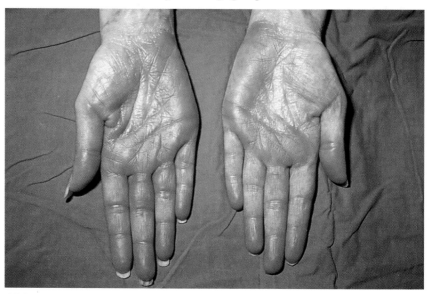

Slide 24

a. What is being shown in this picture?
b. List four causes.

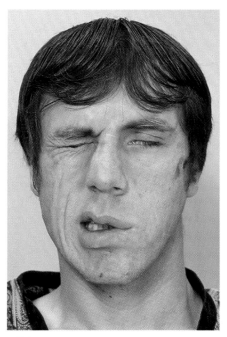

Slide 25

a. What abnormality does this patient manifest?
b. Suggest four possible causes for this appearance.

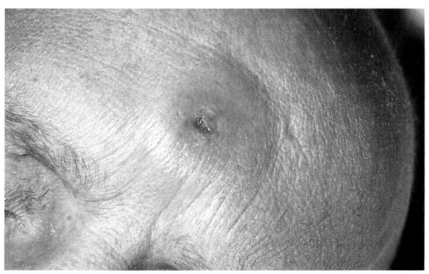

Slide 26

a. What is shown in this neutropenic patient?
b. What is the usual cause for this appearance?

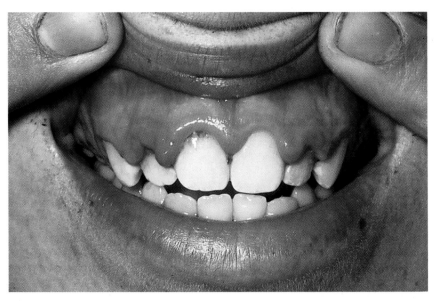

Slide 27

a. What is the abnormality shown?
b. Give four causes for this appearance.
c. What investigation would be helpful?

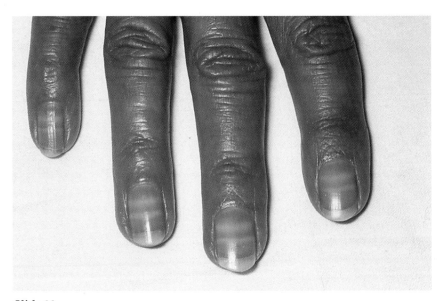

Slide 28

a. What is shown in this picture?
b. What is the likely cause?

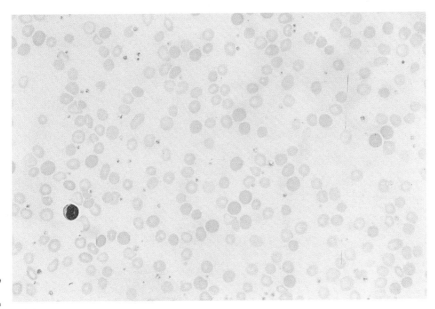

Slide 29

a. List three abnormalities seen on this blood film.
b. Give three conditions giving rise to this appearance.

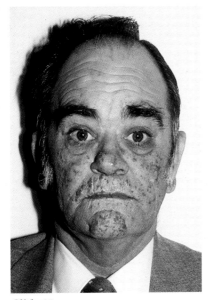

Slide 30

a. What abnormality is demonstrated in this patient?
b. What is the principal complication and its treatment?

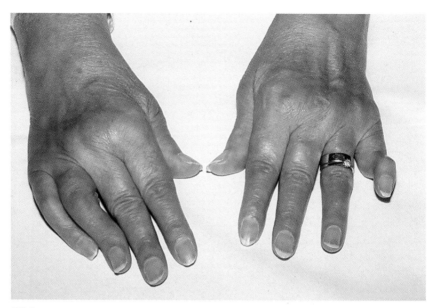

Slide 31

a. Three abnormalities are shown in this picture: list them.
b. Give three haematological complications.

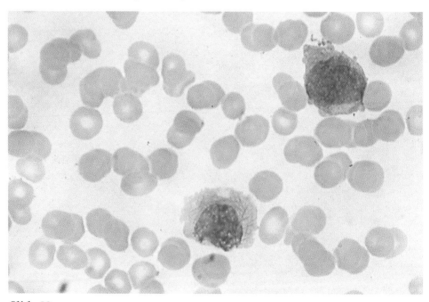

Slide 32

a. What abnormality is shown?
b. What is the underlying condition?

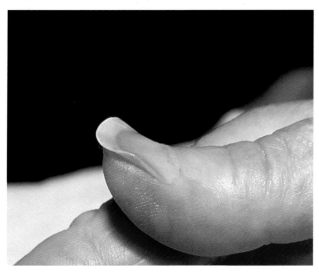

Slide 33

a. What is the abnormality shown?
b. What is the likely underlying basis for this appearance?

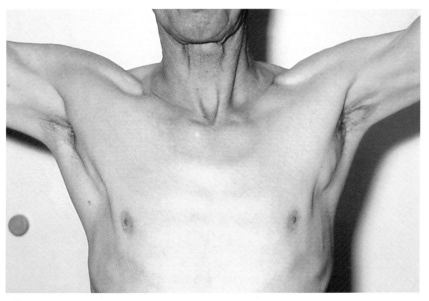

Slide 34

a. What abnormality does this man show?
b. Give three causes for this appearance.
c. What three investigations would you arrange?

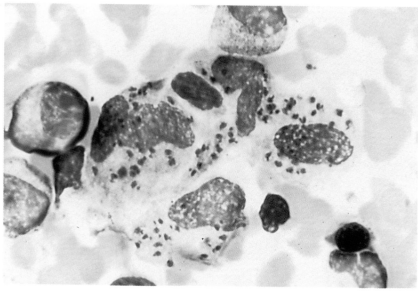

Slide 35

a. What is this preparation?
b. What is the abnormality shown?
c. How would you treat this condition?

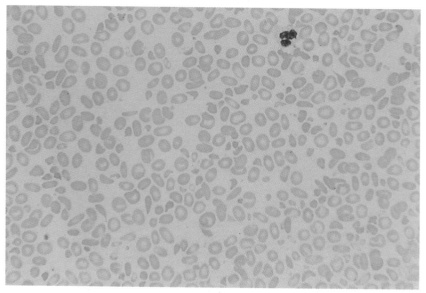

Slide 36

a. Describe this blood film.
b. What is the differential diagnosis?

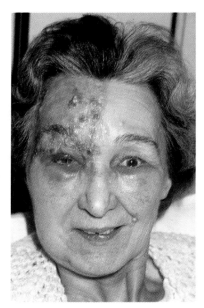

Slide 37

a. What condition is shown in this photograph?
b. Give four complications of this condition.
c. Which haematological diseases typically predispose to this condition?

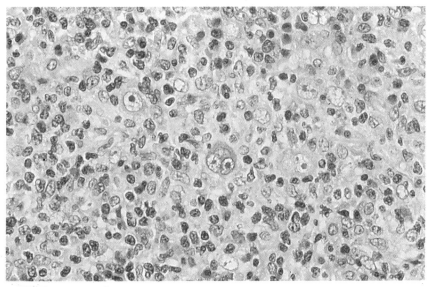

Slide 38

a. What abnormality is shown in this lymph node biopsy?
b. What subtypes of this disease are recognized?

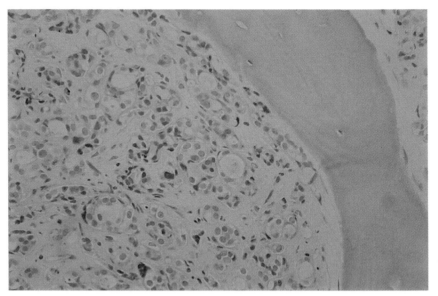

Slide 39

a. Describe the abnormal features in this trephine biopsy.
b. Suggest an underlying cause.

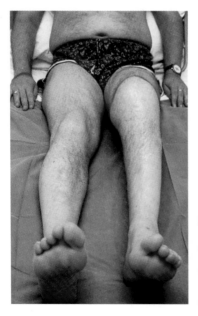

Slide 40

a. What three abnormalities are shown in this picture?
b. What do you think the underlying disorder may be?
c. How would you confirm this?

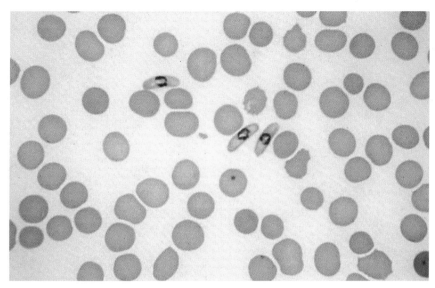

Slide 41

a. Comment on this blood film.
b. Give two serious complications of this disorder.

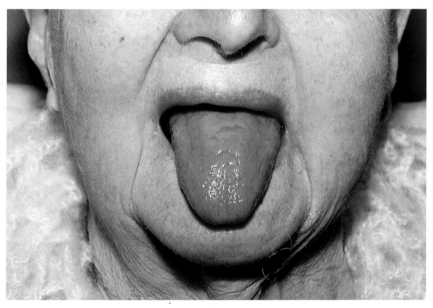

Slide 42

a. Name two abnormalities shown in this picture.
b. What further investigations would you arrange?
c. What complications are associated with this condition?

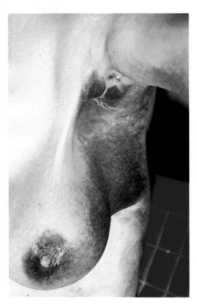

Slide 43

a. Describe the features in this picture.
b. What is the differential diagnosis?
c. What confirmatory tests would you arrange?

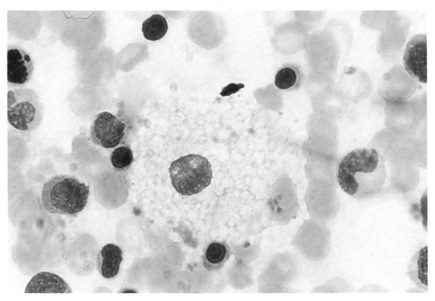

Slide 44

a. What is the abnormality shown?
b. Describe the clinical sequelae.
c. What test would confirm the diagnosis?

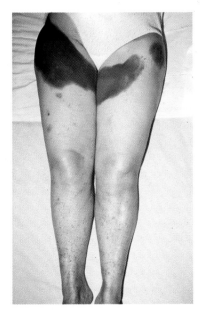

Slide 45

a. Give three causes for this appearance.
b. What investigations would be useful?

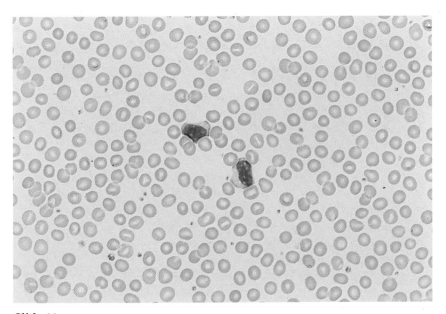

Slide 46

a. Report this peripheral blood film.
b. Give three possible diagnoses.
c. What tests may confirm the diagnosis?

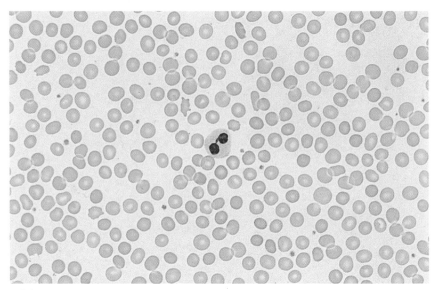

Slide 47

a. What abnormality is shown?
b. What is the underlying disorder?
c. What treatment is available for this disorder?

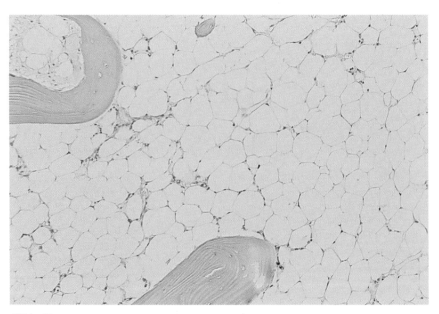

Slide 48

a. Describe the pathological features of this trephine biopsy.
b. Give four causes for this appearance.

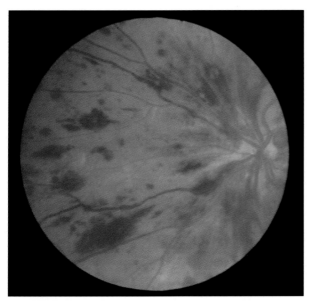

Slide 49

a. Describe three abnormalities in this optic fundus.
b. What is the likely underlying diagnosis and how might it be treated?

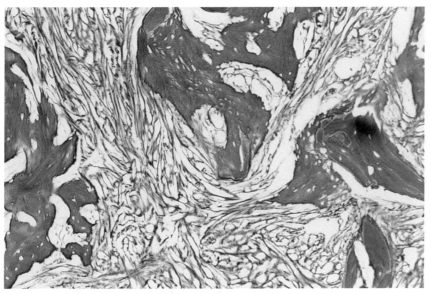

Slide 50

a. What abnormality is shown in this trephine biopsy?
b. What is the likely underlying diagnosis?
c. How would you manage this patient?

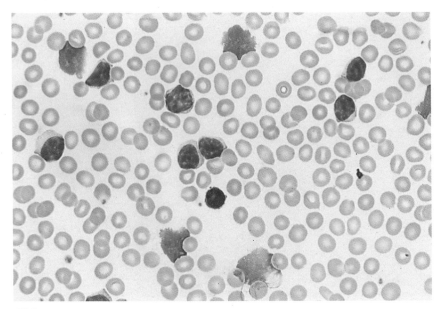

Slide 51

a. What abnormalities are seen on this blood film?
b. What is the likely diagnosis?

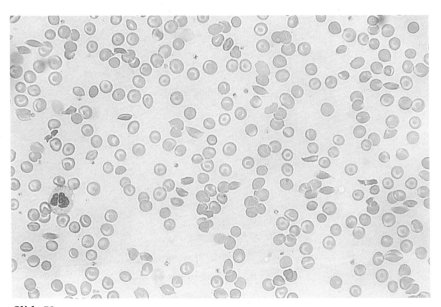

Slide 52

a. List three abnormalities on this peripheral blood film and suggest a diagnosis.
b. Why might this patient limp?

2 Answers to slide questions

Slide 1

a. Lytic lesions scattered throughout the cranium.
b. Multiple myeloma.
Metastatic carcinoma (e.g. lung, breast, thyroid).
Histiocytosis X.
Sarcoidosis.

This patient had multiple myeloma, a disorder of mature B lymphoid cells called plasma cells. Features of the disease include plasma cell accumulation in bone marrow with production of an abnormal paraprotein, typically a monoclonal immunoglobulin, most commonly IgG. Lytic bone lesions and osteoporosis are common, along with renal impairment due to light chain nephropathy. Hyperviscosity symptoms may occur depending on the serum paraprotein level. Other features include anaemia, infection, neurological complications due to nerve compression and peripheral neuropathy secondary to the paraproteinaemia.

> The disease is insidious and by the time of presentation patients often have advanced disease. Treatment consists of chemotherapy, usually with alkylating agents; local radiotherapy is useful for bone pain. Median survival for treated myeloma is 3–4 years. Features associated with the poorest outcome include severe anaemia, hypoalbuminaemia, renal failure, hypercalcaemia and extensive osteolytic lesions.

Multiple myeloma is discussed in the Review articles (Chapter 7).

Final diagnosis
Multiple myeloma.

Slide 2

a. There is balanced translocation between chromosomes 15 and 17, i.e. t(15;17).
b. AML (APML); FAB M3 variant.
c. This is probably the best subgroup of adult AML.

> There are several known non-random karyotypic abnormalities associated with specific neoplastic diseases. These include the Philadelphia chromosome, t(9;22) seen in CML, t(8;21), inv (16), t(15;17) in AML, and t(14;18) in follicular lymphoma.

The t(15;17) is seen in AML M3 (APML). The translocation involves the genes PML and RARα. Remission of the disease has been reported using ATRA alone. However, in order to achieve cure, cytotoxic drugs are required in addition to ATRA.

Final diagnosis

Chromosomal karyotype demonstrating the translocation t(15;17) in APML.

Slide 3

a. Abnormal calcification of the left lung.
   Left-sided pleural effusion.
b. Pulmonary tuberculosis and carcinoma of the lung.

This man was suffering from active tuberculosis, suggested by the ongoing weight loss and shortness of breath. Patients with malignant disease of any type are predisposed to infection, including herpes zoster, tuberculosis and candidiasis. In CLL there is often a secondary hypogammaglobulinaemia which renders these patients particularly immunocompromised. If repeated and/or serious infections occur in CLL, many physicians administer prophylactic IVIg.

Other diseases producing radiographic lesions similar to that found in this patient on CXR include: carcinoma, hamartomas, Wegener's granulomatosis, bronchopulmonary aspergillosis and extrinsic allergic alveolitis.

Final diagnosis

Active tuberculosis in a patient with CLL.

Slide 4

a. The cells are positive for CD19, CD10 and TdT. They are negative for CD14 and CD13. This suggests cALL.
b. Prognostic factors:

	Bad	Good
WBC	$> 50 \times 10^9/l$	$< 10 \times 10^9/l$
Age	< 2 years, ≥ 15 years	2–10 years
Sex	Male	Female
Chromosomes	t(8;14) = L3 subtype t(4;11) = null ALL t(9;22) Hypodiploid	> 50 chromosomes i.e., hyperdiploid
Morphology	FAB subtypes L2 and L3	FAB subtype L1
Markers	B cell (SmIg⁺); T cell	cALL
Others	CNS leukaemia Organomegaly	Remission within 4 weeks

Flow cytometry (often called FACS profile) allows the phenotypic evaluation of around 500 cells per second and enables quantitative assessment of two independent parameters on the same cell; the technology allows evaluation of both cell surface and cytoplasmic antigens and can assist in defining the lineage or pathology of the cells involved. The flow cytometer measures fluorescence and light scatter of cells as they flow in a coaxial stream through a beam of light. The labels used are fluorochromes such as FITC or PE. Using a variety of mirrors, both forward and side scatter of light are measured. Generally, PE is plotted on one axis and FITC on the other. This is demonstrated in Figure 2.1. Gating (i.e. setting the grid lines) refers to the setting of a window through which the electronic events are measured. By observing the population of cells labelled with each fluorochrome and the position relative to the gates, the phenotypic characteristics of the tumour cell population may be determined. Figure 2.1 illustrates this in the following four flow cytometry profiles. The antigens being analysed are A and B and various theoretical combinations of cells are shown to illustrate the point.

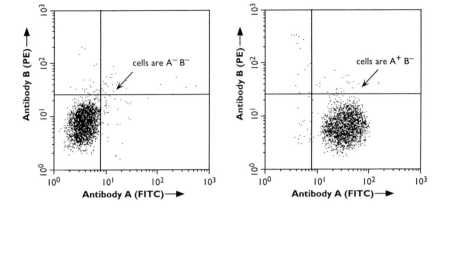

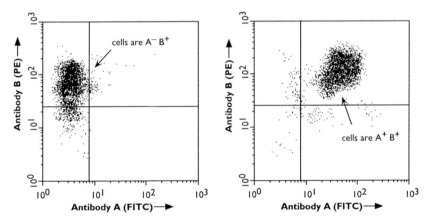

Fig. 2.1   A⁺ B⁺ indicates positive staining for A and B antigens, A⁺ B⁻ indicates positive staining for A antigen but negative staining for B antigen, etc.

Final diagnosis

ALL; flow cytometry profile.

Slide 5

a. Bilateral hilar enlargement.
b. The differential diagnosis is large and includes:

(i) Enlarged lymph nodes:
   – Lymphoma (Hodgkin's disease and non-Hodgkin's lymphoma).
   – Sarcoidosis.
   – Primary tuberculosis.
   – Histoplasmosis.
   – Coccidioidomycosis.
   – Specific infections in childhood (e.g. mycoplasma pneumonia).
(ii) Enlarged blood vessels:
   – Pulmonary arterial hypertension.
   – Left-to-right shunts (atrial or ventricular septal defect, patent ductus arteriosus).

This patient had Hodgkin's disease. Lymphomas classically cause asymmetrical bilateral hilar lymphadenopathy and paratracheal involvement is very common. These appearances contrast with the typical findings in sarcoidosis, where lymph nodes are symmetrically enlarged and paratracheal sites are spared.

Final diagnosis

Hodgkin's disease.

Slide 6

a. Acute lymphoblastic leukaemia.
b. Good.

She has a hyperdiploid karyotype which is associated with good prognosis. Other factors in her favour include: female sex, age (<2 and ≥15 years are bad prognostic group), WBC (>50 × 10^9/l is bad). We are not provided with immunophenotypic data but the best prognosis group is FAB subtype L1 with cALL markers. Other bad prognostic features include: male sex (testicular involvement), translocations t(8;14) associated with L3 subtype, t(9;22), hypodiploid chromosomes, L2 subtype, B- and T cell markers, presence of CNS disease and organomegaly.

Diagnosis

Hyperdiploidy in ALL.

Slide 7

a. A double-contrast barium enema examination. The picture shows the large bowel from mid-transverse colon to rectum.
b. There are multiple diverticula seen in the descending and sigmoid colon.
c. Iron-deficiency anaemia secondary to chronic blood loss.
   Neutrophil leukocytosis and raised ESR during acute episodes of inflammation.

Iron deficiency is usually the result of haemorrhage and the commonest cause on a worldwide basis is probably hookworm infestation. In females of childbearing age menstrual loss is a frequent cause but in men and post-menopausal women iron deficiency is typically due to chronic (and usually occult) blood loss from the GI tract. As a result, radiological or endoscopic investigation of the bowel is central to the management of iron deficiency.

Colonic diverticulosis is a recognized cause of GI bleeding, which is reported in 20–25% cases of diverticular disease. The bleeding tends to be brisk, painless and is not associated with straining.

Final diagnosis

Barium enema with diverticular disease.

Slide 8

a. There is marked widening of the diploic space due to bone marrow hyperplasia. This has resulted in the so-called hair-on-end appearance.
b. β-Thalassaemia major.
c. Iron overload (due to both increased iron absorption and to repeated blood transfusion therapy).
   Ankle ulceration.

The generalized hair-on-end appearance of the skull vault is seen in conditions where there is bone marrow (erythroid) hyperplasia. This generally occurs in the setting of severe chronic anaemic states and there may be associated extramedullary haematopoiesis.

> The most common underlying condition is β-thalassaemia, but it may also be seen in sickle cell anaemia, hereditary spherocytosis and pyruvate kinase deficiency. Similar appearances have also been rarely described in severe iron-deficiency anaemia of childhood and in cyanotic heart disease.

The erythropoietin 'drive' seen in thalassaemia is responsible for the profound marrow expansion, bone thinning, pathological fractures and increased iron absorption characteristic of the thalassaemia syndromes. Skull deformities may lead to sinus and ear infections.

Final diagnosis

β-Thalassaemia major.

Slide 9

a. This is a CXR showing a large mediastinal mass. The lung fields are clear and the cardiac outline is normal.
b. NHL.
   Hodgkin's disease.
   Thymoma.
   Dermoid cyst.
   Teratoma.
   Goitre.
c. CT scan.
   Consider mediastinoscopy and biopsy of mass.
   Bone marrow.
   Cell markers (immunophenotype) on blood and marrow.
   Lactate dehydrogenase.

Mediastinal masses may be anterior, middle or posterior and a lateral CXR is essential in order to define the location more precisely. CT scanning is also very useful to delineate further abnormal masses within the thoracic cavity. The differential diagnosis of a mediastinal mass depends to a large extent on its location.

Adult NHL is the second commonest cause of SVCO after lung carcinoma. Some 3–8% of patients with lymphoma present with SVCO and most will have NHL.

CT is required to gauge the extent of the tumour and plan the biopsy. If there are peripheral lymph nodes, then one of these should be excised for diagnostic purposes. If there are no nodes then mediastinoscopy and biopsy may be required. Bone marrow is required as part of the staging of the lymphoma. LDH is a surrogate marker of disease activity and, again, forms part of the staging procedure. Cell markers provide useful information relating to the cell of origin of the tumour, i.e. B cell, T cell, etc.

Final diagnosis

CXR with mediastinal mass due to high-grade NHL (lymphoblastic NHL).

Slide 10

a. This is an MRI scan (T1-weighted signal) showing a sagittal, midline image of the cervical and thoracic spine. Two discrete soft-tissue masses are present in the mid and lower thoracic regions associated with the vertebral bodies. The upper lesion extends posteriorly into the spinal canal and is seen compressing the spinal cord. The lower lesion lies mainly anterior to the vertebral bodies (extending over three levels) but there is also posterior involvement of the spinal canal and spinal cord compression. The MRI signals from the involved vertebral bodies are abnormal, but in addition, the signals are diffusely abnormal from all the vertebral bodies, suggesting a more generalized bone marrow disorder.

b. Metastatic malignancy – especially those primary tumours that spread to bone:

(i)   Breast.
(ii)   Bronchus.
(iii)   Thyroid.
(iv)   Prostate.
(v)   Kidney.

Multiple myeloma/plasmacytoma.
Lymphoma.
Extramedullary haematopoiesis.

A malignant process is the most likely cause of the appearances shown. This patient presented acutely with signs of spinal cord compression and investigations revealed the presence of multiple soft-tissue plasmacytomas.

> Paraspinal masses consisting of haematopoietic tissue (extramedullary haematopoiesis) are occasionally seen in conditions of severe chronic anaemia or altered bone marrow environment (e.g. β-thalassaemia major or idiopathic myelofibrosis respectively).

Final diagnosis

Multiple plasmacytomas.

Slide 11

a. Large mediastinal mass in the left hemithorax invading the anterior chest wall.
b. Lymphoma.
Carcinoma.

In this patient the cause was high-grade NHL.

> Presentation with mediastinal masses is common in lymphoblastic lymphoma (50–70% of cases) and there may also be associated pleural effusions. Associated symptoms include dyspnoea, dysphagia and pain. If SVCO occurs there is swelling of the neck, face and upper limbs. Lymphadenopathy in the neck, axillae and supraclavicular regions occurs in 50–80% patients. Abdominal involvement is unusual and if it does occur tends to affect the liver and spleen.
>
> If SVCO occurs then DXT is useful to decompress vital structures. Otherwise, chemotherapy should be started to reduce tumour bulk and induce remission.

Final diagnosis

Large mediastinal mass in high-grade NHL/ALL.

Slide 12

a. This patient's marrow cells were predominantly CD33$^+$, CD13$^+$ and MPO$^+$ (i.e. myeloid antigens) and negative for antigens CD3, CD10 and CD19 (lymphoid antigens), suggesting a diagnosis of AML. This was confirmed by morphological, cytochemical and karyotypic analyses.
b. Initial management should consist of treatment of any underlying infection, hydration, and commencing oral allopurinol to prevent tumour lysis syndrome and hyperuricaemia prior to commencing intravenous cytotoxic therapy.

Final diagnosis

AML; flow cytometry profile.

Slide 13

a. Template bleeding time device (Simplate).
b. It is used primarily as a test of platelet function and is indicated if platelet dysfunction is suspected, e.g. thrombasthenia, platelet storage pool diseases, drug or paraprotein-induced platelet dysfunction and myelodysplastic disorders.

Devices such as the one shown have enabled standardization of the bleeding time. The device has either one or two spring-loaded blades which are fired a fixed distance into the skin of the forearm, after which the time taken for bleeding to stop is measured.

The normal range is 3–9 min using standard conditions (supine subject, sphygmomanometer inflated to 40 mmHg, blotting blood flow every 30 s).

Final diagnosis

Template bleeding time device.

Slide 14

a. There are red cell rouleaux. The photograph shows red cells 'stacked up' like piles of coins. This differs from agglutination, which describes a more random clumping of cells.
b. Rouleaux are seen in a variety of clinical situations in which there are increased plasma proteins of high molecular weight, e.g. pregnancy (fibrinogen), multiple myeloma (monoclonal immunoglobulin), and inflammatory disorders (polyclonal immunoglobulins and fibrinogen).
c. Full history and examination for signs of chronic underlying disease, myeloma, etc.
   Serum immunoglobulins and protein electrophoretic strip.
   Autoimmune profile.
   Consider bone marrow aspirate and trephine biopsy.
   C-reactive protein.

Final diagnosis

Red cell rouleaux.

Slide 15

a. Part of the long arm of chromosome 5 is deleted (5q⁻ syndrome).
b. This is associated with MDS.
c. Good, with overall median survival at least 32 months.

The 5q⁻ syndrome is associated with refractory anaemia, hence the lack of response to iron treatment in this patient. This subtype of MDS is particularly found in elderly females in whom a macro-cytic anaemia is often present (hence the trial of vitamin B_{12} and folate). Marrow examination shows marked dyserythropoiesis, erythroid multinuclearity and micromegakaryocytes. Up to 50% of patients have splenomegaly and the platelet count is normal or increased.

> The 5q⁻ breakpoint involves haematopoietic growth factor genes, including IL-3, IL-4, IL-5, M-CSF, GM-CSF and the c-fms proto-oncogene (the M-CSF receptor).

Final diagnosis

Chromosomal karyotype demonstrating the 5q⁻ abnormality in MDS.

Slide 16

a. This is a Southern blot showing hybridization of the JH probe to complementary sequences in the digested control DNA as well as the DNA from the 3 patients. The final result, as shown in this photograph, is an autoradiograph.
b. Patients 1 and 3 show identical patterns to that of the normal control, suggesting that these patients do not appear to have a clonal B cell population (e.g. as found in B-CLL). Patient 2, however, has a band in a different position to the control. This is termed a rearranged or non-germline band and supports the diagnosis of B-CLL.

> Southern blotting has been used for several years to detect clonal gene rearrangements in human malignant cells. A number of gene probes are available that allow detection of altered immunoglobulin, T cell receptor genes and other loci. The principle involves digestion of DNA from patients' blood or marrow samples. The digested DNA is then subjected to agarose gel electrophoresis which separates fragments on the basis of size (cf. globin electrophoresis, where proteins are separated on the basis of electrical charge). In order to detect the digested

fragments of the immunoglobulin gene a known probe is used which, after radiolabelling, is detected by exposing the patient DNA with hybridized probe to X-ray film, thus generating the autoradiograph. The location of the labelled fragment is seen as a dark band and is well demonstrated in this picture.

Since the rearranged band in patient 2 has travelled a shorter distance than the control band this implies that the immunoglobulin gene fragment of the patient is larger than that of the control DNA.

Final diagnosis

B cell lymphoid neoplasm; clonality demonstrated by Southern blotting.

Slide 17

a. Isoelectric focusing of haemoglobin.

> A similar pattern would have been obtained using cellulose acetate electrophoresis but the bands shown in Slide 17 are well defined in keeping with IEF. Haemoglobins migrate to characteristic positions on the IEF gel, a technique that allows accurate identification of abnormal haemoglobins that cannot be separated or identified using other techniques, e.g. citrate agar. Another advantage of IEF gels is the ability to run large numbers of samples simultaneously making it highly suitable for haemoglobinopathy screening programmes.

b. Patients 1 and 2 have HbC trait (they each have haemoglobin A and C). Patient 3 is normal (haemoglobin A only) and patient 4 has sickle cell trait (AS).

c. Since they are both AC, they have a 25% chance of having a child with AA (normal), a 50% chance of having a child with AC (HbC trait) and 25% chance of having a child with HbC disease.

d. This couple has a 25% chance of having a child with AA (normal), AS (sickle trait), AC (HbC trait) or HbSC.

> HbSC produces a similar, but milder, disease to sickle cell disease (HbSS) but patients may still suffer crises. Proliferative retinopathy occurs in SS but is considerably worse in SC disease. The haemolysis in SC is less than that seen in SS. HbC disease is a β globin abnormality in which the glutamic acid at position 6 is replaced by lysine. The red cells are more rigid than normal and HbC crystals may form within red blood cells. Red cell life span is reduced. Clinical features include splenomegaly and mild anaemia (Hb ~8–12 g/dl). Target cells are prominent in the peripheral blood film. Unlike sickle cell anaemia and SC disease, HbC disease is a relatively mild disorder.

Final diagnosis

HbA, AS, AC.

Slide 18

a. CLL (CD19$^+$, CD5$^+$, κ$^+$).
b. CLL is one of the low-grade lymphoproliferative disorders. Most cases are due to B cell expansion, hence the CD19 positivity. CD5 is a T cell marker that is aberrantly expressed in CLL, distinguishing it from other B cell lymphoid malignancies such as HCL, follicular lymphoma, etc.
The disorder is associated with a long natural history dependent upon the presence of marrow failure, lymphadenopathy, splenomegaly and other features.

CLL is discussed fully in the Review articles (Chapter 7).

Final diagnosis

CLL; flow cytometry profile.

Slide 19

a. Radioisotope bone scan.
b. 'Hot spots' in skull.
c. Bone metastases.

Radioisotope bone scanning is performed by injecting technetium (^{99}Tc^m, in pertechnetate form) intravenously. This radiochemical is useful for providing static brain studies. Following i.v. injection the radiochemical equilibrates with the extracellular fluid and does not penetrate the blood/brain barrier. Normal brain structures are therefore not visualized. Instead the agent is useful for demonstrating abnormalities affecting the vasculature or processes that *destroy* the blood/brain barrier. ^{99}Tc^m is safe, carries little radiation dose and may be used for outpatient investigation.

The appearances here suggest likely metastases from breast, lung or prostate. This form of scanning is not useful in the diagnosis of multiple myeloma (the skeletal survey involving plain radiology should be performed).

Final diagnosis

Bone scan demonstrating 'hot spots' in skull.

Slide 20

a. There is a well-defined stricture of the descending colon producing a typical 'apple-core' lesion.
b. Carcinoma of the large intestine.
c. Anaemia:
  (i)   iron-deficient (bleeding).
  (ii) microangiopathic (secondary to underlying cancer).
  (iii) leukoerythroblastic (infiltration of the marrow by metastases).
  (iv) anaemia of chronic disorders.
  Disseminated intravascular coagulation.
  Bleeding if there is hepatic dysfunction secondary to underlying liver metastases.
  Bleeding secondary to presence of acquired clotting factor deficiency.

Final diagnosis

Carcinoma of the colon shown on barium enema.

Slide 21

a. CML in chronic phase.
b. The main complication is transformation from chronic (i.e. stable phase) CML to a more acute (and aggressive) leukaemic phase. This is generally acute myeloid leukaemic transformation but in some instances takes the form of acute lymphoid leukaemia. Other complications include priapism, leukostatic syndrome and secondary hyperuricaemia.

CML is a stem cell disorder characterized by a predominance of granulocytic cells in blood and marrow. This blood film shows the usual features of chronic phase CML with large numbers of immature and mature granulocytic cells (e.g. neutrophils and their precursors). In chronic phase the blast cell (i.e. immature cell) number is low. Peripheral blood basophilia is common.

> This disorder is associated with the Philadelphia chromosome, a balanced translocation between chromosomes 9 and 22. This was the first non-random chromosome abnormality shown to be associated with a specific neoplasm and was described by Nowell and Hungerford in 1960. In the translocation c-abl on chromosome 9 is joined to bcr on chromosome 22, generating a chimeric bcr-abl gene whose product is a novel p210 bcr-abl protein (Fig. 2.2).

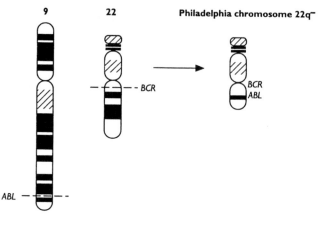

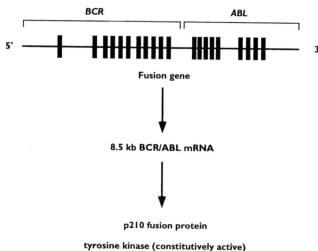

Fig. 2.2   Philadelphia chromosome: cytogenetic and molecular features

The presence of the Philadelphia chromosome may be confirmed using standard cytogenetic analysis, Southern blotting or PCR amplification of the bcr-abl mRNA (using a reverse transcriptase PCR assay). The p210 protein, a tyrosine kinase, has been shown to be central to the dysregulation of haematopoiesis seen in CML.

The Philadelphia chromosome is present in 90–95% of patients with CML. The remainder of patients have variant translocations or molecular abnormalities of the long arm of chromosome 22.

After 3–5 years the disease may undergo an accelerated phase with transformation to an acute blastic phase with the emergence of acute (usually myeloid) leukaemia. Even with appropriate chemotherapy the acute leukaemia often responds poorly and the outlook is fairly bleak. The best therapeutic option for younger patients with CML is sibling allogeneic BMT whilst in chronic phase. Transplants carried out in acute blast transformation offer little hope of cure and relapse is early in comparison to transplants carried out in chronic phase where the remission is longer and there is a realistic chance of cure.

Recent trials show that interferon-α treatment is capable of prolonging survival in CML.

Reference

Nowell, P.C. and Hungerford, D.A. (1960) A minute chromosome in human granulocytic leukemia. *Science* **132**, 1497.

Final diagnosis

Chronic phase CML.

Slide 22

a. This elderly woman with lymphoma has oral candidiasis affecting predominantly the tongue.
b. Oral candidiasis (thrush) can occur in immunocompromised patients with disorders such as diabetes mellitus, carcinoma, alcoholism and cachexia. *Candida* species are the commonest cause of fungal infection in immunocompromised patients.

Lymphoreticular malignancies such as acute and chronic leukaemias also predispose to this infection. Patients receiving chemotherapy rendering them neutropenic are also at particular risk, as are patients receiving a variety of antibacterial agents. HIV infection is also a well-recognized cause of candidiasis.

The agent is *Candida albicans*, a yeast normally found throughout the GI tract. When host defences are reduced, through illness or drugs, this normal commensal grows freely, producing the characteristic white monilial patches on the oral mucosa and tongue.

Oral infections usually respond well to agents such as fluconazole or nystatin suspension. Systemic candidal infection is a serious disorder that may involve lungs, kidneys, heart, brain and/or liver and requires treatment with i.v. amphotericin B.

Final diagnosis

Oral candidiasis in a patient with CLL.

Slide 23

a. There is a total absence of platelets in this film. The red cells are normal; the film shows a solitary neutrophil which also looks quite normal.

b. ITP.

There are two separate forms of this disorder: childhood and adult. The childhood type is often preceded by a viral infection, followed by acute thrombocytopenia which commonly requires no treatment and resolves spontaneously, usually within 4 weeks. The adult form often has no prodromal illness and is a chronic remitting and relapsing condition which usually requires treatment with corticosteroids.

> Second-line treatments include IVIg or splenectomy. ITP is associated with the presence of antiplatelet antibodies (IgG) which are autoantibodies arising 'spontaneously' or following viral infections. In both forms there is premature removal of antibody-coated platelets by the reticuloendothelial system. Mucosal bleeding is prominent in both types and this often takes the form of epistaxes, gum bleeding, bruising and purpura.

ITP is discussed in the Review articles (Chapter 7).

Final diagnosis

ITP.

Slide 24

a. Palmar erythema.

b. Liver disease, rheumatoid arthritis, pregnancy, thyrotoxicosis, subacute bacterial endocarditis, chronic febrile illness and GVHD.

GVHD is seen in allogeneic transplantation wherein immunocompetent donor T cells react against tissues of the recipient of the graft. Characteristic features include fever, liver dysfunction, diarrhoea and skin rashes.

The skin rash involves particularly the palms and soles but other areas of the body are also affected. Following an erythematous phase there is eventual epidermolysis and exfoliation of affected areas.

Although by no means pathognomonic, the intensely erythematous palms in this patient who has undergone sibling donor BMT does suggest GVHD. In fact, the patient had other stigmata suggesting this diagnosis.

Prevention involves the use of methotrexate and cyclosporin immunosuppression. Other measures involve donor T cell depletion, but this reduces the graft-versus-leukaemia effect of the transplant. If GVHD occurs, treatment includes the use of high-dose i.v. methylprednisolone.

Final diagnosis

GVHD producing palmar erythema.

Slide 25

a. Left lower motor neurone seventh (facial) nerve palsy.
b. Meningeal malignancy (leukaemia, lymphoma or carcinoma).
   Space-occupying lesions of the cerebellopontine angle.
   Herpes zoster infections of the geniculate ganglion (Ramsay Hunt syndrome).
   Bell's palsy (idiopathic).
   Tumours involving the parotid.
   Mononeuropathy as part of systemic disease (e.g. diabetes mellitus or sarcoidosis).

The patient had been asked to show his teeth and screw up his eyelids. The obvious weakness of the left upper and lower facial muscles is characteristic. This appearance is different from an upper motor neurone lesion, where there is relative preservation of power in the muscles of the upper part of the face. This is because the upper facial muscles are bilaterally innervated from the cerebral hemispheres.

This patient had ALL with meningeal leukaemic infiltration. Lumbar puncture revealed leukaemic blast cells present in the cerebrospinal fluid. CNS involvement is a common feature of high-grade lymphoid malignancies (ALL, lymphoblastic lymphoma, immunoblastic lymphoma). It is generally a poor prognostic feature as treatment is often unsatisfactory, with poor disease control. As a result of this, CNS prophylactic treatment is usually part of the management of these aggressive haematological malignancies, when they present without overt CNS involvement.

Final diagnosis

Seventh nerve palsy due to CNS involvement with ALL.

Slide 26

a. Ecthyma gangrenosum. There is the characteristic lesion on this patient's forehead consisting of a central necrotic bulla surrounded by a thin band of erythema.

b. Gram-negative septicaemia, most commonly associated with *Pseudomonas aeruginosa*. Ecthyma gangrenosum is seen in about 5% of patients with *Pseudomonas* sepsis in the setting of granulocytopenia or severe immunosuppression. The lesions may be single or multiple and occur most often on the legs, abdomen, axillae and anogenital areas. Other Gram-negative organisms can be associated, such as *Aeromonas hydrophilia*, *Klebsiella* spp., *Escherichia coli* and *Proteus* spp.

> The differential diagnosis of these lesions includes fungal septicaemia due to *Candida* spp., pyoderma gangrenosum, necrotizing vasculitis, cryoglobulinaemia, hyperviscosity syndrome and leukaemic infiltrates.

Final diagnosis

Ecthyma gangrenosum in a neutropenic patient.

Slide 27

a. Hypertrophy of the gums.
b. Causes of gum hypertrophy include:
   (i)   Drugs, especially phenytoin and cyclosporin. Gingival hyperplasia has also been reported with nifedipine and oral contraceptives.
   (ii) Acute myelomonocytic leukaemia.
   (iii) Chronic myelomonocytic leukaemia.
   (iv) Scurvy.
   (v)   Pregnancy.
c. If no drug cause or dietary insufficiency is apparent then an FBC and film should be performed.

Final diagnosis

Acute myelomonocytic leukaemia with associated gum hypertrophy.

Slide 28

a. Beau's lines. All the nails show multiple white transverse lines. These are spaced regularly on the nails in both the horizontal and vertical directions.
b. Interruption of nail growth during repeated cycles of intensive cytotoxic chemotherapy.

   Beau's lines represent a transient interference in the growth pattern of the nails. When isolated to one nail, local injury is the likely cause. When all the nails are affected, these indicate recent systemic illness (such as severe infections, coronary thrombosis, etc.). When the upset has been severe, the Beau's lines can result in ridging of the nails. The effect of a course of chemotherapy usually stops short of ridging but causes a characteristic whitening of the nail texture. The striking appearance here reflects sequential courses of intensive chemotherapy and the nails provide a temporal record of each course, rather like the rings of a tree trunk.

Final diagnosis

Beau's lines caused by cytotoxic chemotherapy.

Slide 29

a. This film shows dimorphic red blood cells: there are clearly two populations of cells – smaller pale cells with larger cells containing relatively greater amounts of haemoglobin.
b. Dimorphic red cells may be seen:
   (i)   Following recent blood transfusion.
   (ii) In iron deficiency when therapy has been recently commenced and when there is an adequate response.
   (iii) In primary acquired sideroblastic anaemia, one of the milder forms of myelodysplasia.

Final diagnosis

Dimorphic blood film.

Slide 30

a. This man has multiple telangiectases affecting the skin on his face and lips.
b. These lesions bleed and because they are often scattered throughout the GI tract, blood loss may be substantial. The main complication is iron-deficiency anaemia.

This man has Osler–Weber–Rendu syndrome (hereditary haemorrhagic telangiectasia) which is an autosomal dominant condition resulting in abnormalities of the elastic fibres of the small vessels affecting skin, mucous membranes and many internal organs. These lesions characteristically blanch on pressure (cf. purpura). Nose and gum bleeding is common and the condition often worsens with advancing age since the vascular abnormalities become worse. Arteriovenous fistulae in the lungs may develop and cause massive haemoptysis.

Treatment includes oral or i.v. iron replacement therapy, blood transfusions, systemic oestrogen therapy or surgery/cautery to local bleeding points.

Final diagnosis

Hereditary haemorrhagic telangiectasia (Osler–Weber–Rendu syndrome).

Slide 31

a. There is ulnar deviation of the fingers, swelling of the meta-carpophalangeal joints, 'swan neck' deformity and boutonnière deformity. This patient has RA.
b. RA is associated with a number of complications, some directly due to the disease, others reflecting problems in treatment. Clinical diagnosis of the precise complication can be difficult.

Commoner problems include:
  (i) Secondary, chronic disorder anaemia: this may present with a significantly reduced MCV in some 30% of cases. This may be confused with:
  (ii) Iron deficiency anaemia: usually the result of GI blood loss from non-steroidal anti-inflammatory drugs.
  (iii) Autoimmune haemolysis: occasionally a warm antibody autoimmune haemolytic anaemia can develop.
  (iv) Oxidative haemolysis: in sensitive individuals receiving treatment with oxidative drugs such as dapsone.

(v)   Macrocytosis: reflecting treatment with azathioprine or methotrexate.

(vi)   Leukopenia: neutropenia as an idiosyncratic reaction to drug treatment
   – dose-related, reflecting immunosuppressive/cytotoxic therapy.
   – an autoimmune effect.

(vii) Thrombocytopenia:
   – autoimmune.
   – drug-related.
   – due to hypersplenism.

(viii) Pancytopenia: Felty's   syndrome,   associated   with splenomegaly.

Final diagnosis

Rheumatoid disease; haematological complications.

Slide 32

a. This is a bone marrow examination showing numerous heavily granulated promyelocytes containing many Auer rods arranged as bundles, hence the term 'faggot cells'.

b. This is pathognomonic of APML (FAB subtype M3).

APML accounts for ~10–15% of all cases of AML. Approximately 90% of patients have a bleeding diathesis at presentation and cerebral haemorrhage is an important cause of death during remission induction. It is thought to arise from the release of plasminogen activators from the leukaemic granules activating the fibrinolytic pathway.

> Most cases of APML have a characteristic cytogenetic abnormality with translocation of DNA between chromosomes 15 and 17, i.e. t(15;17)(q22;q21): this is shown in Figure 2.3. The breakpoint on chromosome 17 encodes the RARα, whilst the PML gene is located on chromosome 15. The resultant fusion protein (PML/RARα) contains functional domains in both PML and RARα and binds ATRA. The fusion protein thus acts as an ATRA-dependent transcription factor. It has been shown that the fusion protein PML/RARα is responsible for the differentiation block characteristic of APML. The role of the retinoic acid receptor gene in the pathogenesis of APML has led to the discovery that ATRA, which induces differentiation of the leukaemic cells, may, alone, achieve remission in 80% of *de novo* cases of APML.
>
> The effects of retinoids are mediated by two classes of retinoic acid receptor: RARs and RXRs. RARs and RXRs are both members of a superfamily of related ligand-inducible transcriptional regulatory factors. RARs (α, β and γ) are activated by ATRA and 9-*cis* retinoic acid. RXRs (α, β and γ) are activated by 9-*cis* retinoic acid only.

Final diagnosis

APML (AML M3).

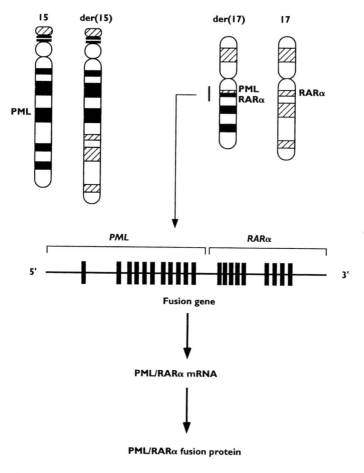

Fig. 2.3   t(15;17) in M3 acute myeloid leukaemia

Slide 33

a. The nail bed appears concave with consequent 'spooning' of the nails. This is the classical appearance of koilonychia.
b. Koilonychia is associated with iron-deficiency anaemia.

Koilonychia, angular stomatitis and mild glossitis are commonly described signs of iron deficiency. They usually reflect chronic deficiency but are not of major diagnostic significance. Clinical management necessitates proving iron deficiency by biochemical or haematological testing, giving iron replacement and determining the cause.

Atrophy of the skin occurs in roughly 30% of patients and nail changes such as koilonychia (spoon-shaped nails) result in brittle flattened nails. Patients may also complain of angular stomatitis in which painful cracks appear at the angle of the mouth, along with glossitis. Further, oesophageal and pharyngeal webs may develop (consider in middle-aged women presenting with dysphagia). It is felt that these changes are due to a reduction in the iron-containing enzymes within the epithelium and GI tract.

Final diagnosis

Iron deficiency anaemia; koilonychia.

Slide 34

a. This man has bilateral axillary lymphadenopathy.
b. The causes of lymphadenopathy include:
   (i) Neoplastic disease (e.g. lymphoma, CLL).
   (ii) Infection (e.g. infectious mononucleosis, HIV seroconversion, CMV, tuberculosis).
   (iii) Autoimmune disease (e.g. SLE, rheumatoid).
   (iv) Sarcoidosis.
c. FBC and film may be informative. Viral titres, cell surface markers and autoantibodies should be checked. One of the lymph nodes should be biopsied.

Final diagnosis

CLL with bilateral axillary lymphadenopathy.

Slide 35

a. Bone marrow aspirate film stained with May–Grünwald–Giemsa stain.
b. There are several macrophages containing Leishman–Donovan bodies. The diagnosis is visceral leishmaniasis or kala-azar.
c. Pentavalent antimalarial drugs remain the mainstay of therapy. Refractory cases may respond to amphotericin B (especially liposomal formulations) or pentamidine.

Infection with the protozoan *Leishmania donovani* is transmitted by the bite of the female sandfly, *Phlebotomus*. The reservoir of infection is the amastigote form of the parasite, present in animal hosts such as rodents, dogs and foxes or in humans. There is a variable incubation period from a few months to several years and the typical presentation is with gradual onset of fever, debility, weight loss, hepatosplenomegaly and pancytopenia. Polyclonal increases in immunoglobulins (chiefly IgG) are also characteristic.

Diagnosis is usually made by examining splenic aspirates, bone marrow aspirate or tissue biopsies for the characteristic amastigotes (intracellular Leishman–Donovan bodies).

Kala-azar is distributed mainly throughout tropical and warm regions of the world. It is present around the Mediterranean basin and hence may be acquired by holiday-makers to that area.

Final diagnosis

Kala-azar; Leishman–Donovan bodies demonstrated in marrow macrophages.

Slide 36

a. The red cells appear quite abnormal. There is gross anisopoikilocytosis and the red cells have surface projections.
b. Iron deficiency, megaloblastic anaemia, myelofibrosis, pyruvate kinase deficiency, HPP.

   This film is characteristic of HPP, a congenital haemolytic anaemia with autosomal recessive inheritance. It shares features with hereditary elliptocytosis. The term is derived from the *in vitro* phenomenon of red cell fragmentation on heating which occurs at lower temperatures than that seen with normal red cells.

> In some cases a spectrin defect is the underlying cause.
> Polyacrylamide gel electrophoresis reveals a partial defect of spectrin with decreased spectrin : band 3 ratio.
> The differential diagnosis includes iron deficiency, thalassaemias, megaloblastic anaemia, myelofibrosis, myelodysplasia and pyruvate kinase deficiency.

No treatment is required if the disorder is mild. In severe cases splenectomy may be of value and, in some patients, life-saving.

Final diagnosis

Hereditary pyropoikilocytosis.

Slide 37

a. Herpes zoster involving the ophthalmic division of the right trigeminal nerve (Va)–herpes zoster ophthalmicus.

b. Conjunctivitis, keratitis, iridocyclitis.
Optic neuritis occasionally occurs.
Associated cranial nerve involvement (typically VII, with facial palsy).
Encephalomyelitis.
Secondary bacterial infection (streptococcal, staphylococcal).
Dissemination (in immunocompromised patients).
Post-herpetic neuralgia.

c. Chronic (low-grade) lymphoproliferative disorders, especially CLL.

Herpes zoster is a frequent cause of morbidity in patients with CLL and may present in any dermatome or cranial nerve root. The underlying cause is the acquired immune deficiency (both hypogammaglobulinaemia and cellular immune defects) produced by the disease. Such patients are particularly vulnerable to the complications of zoster listed above, and they should be treated promptly with antiviral drugs and appropriate supportive care. Systemic acyclovir or oral valaciclovir are the agents of choice, but should be started at, or soon after, the onset of symptoms and signs to be effective. Given later, they may still truncate the course of the infection and, in particular, may prevent dissemination. There is also a role for acyclovir in the prevention of recurrence and in prophylaxis against herpes zoster infections in these immunocompromised patients.

Final diagnosis

Herpes zoster affecting trigeminal nerve (Va) in immunocompromised patient.

Slide 38

a. There is a pleomorphic cellular infiltrate including a typical giant binucleate Reed–Sternberg cell and several mononuclear Hodgkin's cells. The diagnosis is Hodgkin's disease of mixed cellularity subtype.

b. Lymphocyte-predominant.
Mixed cellularity.
Nodular sclerosing.
Lymphocyte-depleted.

The Reed–Sternberg cell is not diagnostic of Hodgkin's disease in isolation and can indeed be found in other disease processes such as NHL. Rather, Hodgkin's disease should be regarded as a neoplasm of lymphoid tissue defined histopathologically by Reed–Sternberg cells in the appropriate cellular background. It is the mixture of benign, reactive cells and the neoplastic cells which sets it apart from most other lymphomas.

The cellular origin of the Reed–Sternberg cell remains unknown, but it is thought to represent a highly abnormal activated B or T lymphocyte. It typically expresses only a few B or T cell-associated antigens and is negative for CD45 (leukocyte common antigen). However, it expresses CD30 (Ki-1) and CD15 (Leu-M1).

The Rye classification of Hodgkin's disease recognizes four histological subtypes (listed above), distinguished on the basis of the appearance of the relative proportions of Reed–Sternberg cells, lymphocytes and fibrosis. The histology does have prognostic significance, with lymphocyte predominance being most favourable and lymphocyte depletion least favourable. However, the anatomical extent or stage of the disease is also a key factor in the clinical features, prognosis and optimal management of Hodgkin's disease.

Final diagnosis

Reed–Sternberg cell – Hodgkin's disease.

Slide 39

a. The marrow architecture is highly abnormal with reduction of the normal marrow elements and infiltration by non-haematopoietic cells. There are several groups of cells arranged in gland-like structures.
b. Infiltration of the bone marrow by carcinoma, most likely adenocarcinoma.

Possible primary sites include:
(i) Breast.
(ii) Prostate.
(iii) Large bowel.
(iv) Stomach.

In bone marrow infiltration by tumours there may be focal or diffuse infiltration with variable degrees of fibrosis. Fibrosis is a prominent feature of infiltration by cancers of the breast, prostate, lung and stomach.

To confirm the diagnosis, specific monoclonal antibodies may be used to stain haematopoietic and non-haematopoietic tissue. For example, blood cells may be stained with anti-CD45 (leukocyte common antigen), whereas epithelial antigens may be stained using specific monoclonal antibodies. Adenocarcinoma may be confirmed by staining for mucin.

Adenocarcinomas metastasizing to bone marrow include breast, renal, prostate, GI tract tumours, ovary, endometrium and pancreas.

It is important to identify prostate and breast primary tumours since many cases are responsive to hormonal therapy.

Final diagnosis

Metastatic carcinoma involving the bone marrow; primary site prostate.

Slide 40

a. Swelling of the left knee.
   Fixed flexion deformity of the left knee joint.
   Wasting of the left calf muscles.
b. These appearances, in a male patient, are very characteristic of haemophilia (A or B).
c. A coagulation screen should be performed. Both haemophilia A and B (Christmas disease) cause the APTT to be prolonged. The abnormality is corrected by the addition of normal plasma. The PT and TT are normal, as is the bleeding time.

Assays of levels of FVIII and FIX will establish the diagnosis and severity and will distinguish between haemophilia A and B.

The knee joint should be X-rayed as haemophilic arthropathy has characteristic radiological appearances.

> Haemophilia A and B are the commonest inherited disorders of coagulation factors. Apart from FXI deficiency (which has a high incidence among Ashkenazi Jews, and in which haemarthrosis is very rare), all other coagulation factor deficiencies are exceedingly uncommon.
>
> von Willebrand's disease is associated with reduced levels of FVIII but the major clinical manifestation is mucocutaneous bleeding, and haemarthrosis is not usually seen.

Final diagnosis

Haemophilic arthropathy in a patient with haemophilia A.

Slide 41

a. This thin blood film (stained with May–Grünwald–Giemsa) shows the crescentic gametocytes of *Plasmodium falciparum*.
b. Cerebral malaria.
   Blackwater fever.

When examining a slide for malaria the first aim is to determine the presence or absence of parasites. The next priority in the identification of parasites is whether *Plasmodium falciparum* is present as this is the only one of the four species of human malaria that may constitute a medical emergency. In this regard, the banana-shaped gametocyte of *P. falciparum* is quite unmistakable so, if seen, the diagnosis is immediately established. Gametocytes are often seen persisting in the blood for some 1–2 weeks following successful treatment of the malaria. Other morphological pointers to *P. falciparum* are a high level of parasitaemia (>5%) and the presence of two or more rings within the same red blood cell.

Cerebral malaria is the most lethal complication of *P. falciparum* malaria. It tends to occur only in non-immune subjects but the pathogenesis remains unclear. Localized disturbance of the intracerebral circulation by parasitized red cells seems likely as the brain capillaries often appear to be obstructed by schizonts in fatal cases. Disturbances of consciousness or fits are common presenting features and, if untreated, there is usually progression to coma and death.

Blackwater fever is a syndrome associated with *P. falciparum* infection, when severe intravascular haemolysis is associated with haemoglobinuria and renal failure. It is now seen very rarely.

Final diagnosis

Gametocytes of *Plasmodium falciparum*.

Slide 42

a. Smooth tongue and angular cheilitis.
b. Serum vitamin B_{12} and folate assays.
c. Anaemia, leukopenia, thrombocytopenia, neurological complications.

The diagnosis here was vitamin B_{12} deficiency. Vitamin B_{12}, in conjunction with folate, is required for DNA synthesis. Laboratory features of B_{12} deficiency include oval macrocytosis, marked anisopoikilocytosis, Howell–Jolly bodies (nuclear remnants) and Cabot's rings. Circulating erythroblasts are occasionally seen on the blood film. Reticulocytes are low and neutrophils show hyper-segmentation (nuclei of >5% neutrophils have >5 lobes). Biochemistry screening will show elevated LDH and bilirubin. Examination of the marrow will show erythroid hyperplasia with megaloblastic changes in red cells (haemoglobinized red cells with immature nuclei, nuclear/cytoplasmic asynchrony).

The neurological complications of B_{12} deficiency include paraesthesiae in the fingers and toes, disturbance of position and vibration. Untreated, the disorder may progress to ataxia due to demyelination of posterior and lateral columns (subacute combined degeneration of the cord).

The indices and blood film features of B_{12} and folate deficiency are indistinguishable.

Final diagnosis

Vitamin B_{12} or folate deficiency.

Slide 43

a. This is an elderly female with severe bruising affecting her left arm and breast.
b. The differential diagnosis is wide and should include any disorder associated with reduced platelets or abnormal coagulation. The more likely diagnoses are:
  (i)   Trauma.
  (ii) DIC.
  (iii) ITP.
  (iv) TTP.
  (v)   Acquired FVIII inhibitor.
c. FBC, film and coagulation screen should be performed.

This woman had an acquired FVIII inhibitor. This is the most common form of acquired autoantibodies to coagulation factors but is still rare, affecting approximately 1 per 1 000 000 people per year.

Most patients are over 50 years of age and 50% have an underlying autoimmune disorder. The condition has also been associated with underlying malignancy. Patients often present with large ecchymoses and have a prolonged APTT that does not correct with the addition of normal plasma (cf. factor deficiency).

Most patients with an autoantibody respond to immunosuppressive therapy with prednisolone or cyclophosphamide. A response to IVIg has been reported.

Final diagnosis

Acquired FVIII inhibitor.

Slide 44

a. This bone marrow aspirate shows a large histiocytic cell with foamy cytoplasmic deposits due to lipid accumulation. The appearances are typical of Niemann–Pick disease.
b. In the best-defined form of Niemann–Pick disease (type I) there is an inherited deficiency of the enzyme sphingomyelinase and sphingomyelin accumulates in the body tissues. However, there is a wide clinical spectrum ranging from acute neuropathic forms, presenting in infancy to chronic non-neuropathic forms presenting in early adult life. The predominant features are hepatosplenomegaly and mild lymphadenopathy. In addition, there is often a fine xanthomatous rash. Neurological involvement, when present, can result in seizures, ophthalmoplegia and psychomotor retardation.
c. Demonstration of sphingomyelinase deficiency in leukocytes or in cultured fibroblasts.

Niemann–Pick disease is one of the lipid storage disorders and, in the classical type I disease, the genetic basis is well defined. Inheritance is autosomal recessive and the disorder, although rare, is common among Ashkenazi Jews. Extensive storage of sphingomyelin results in hepatic and splenic enlargement and the characteristic foam cells that are seen in the bone marrow.

There is no effective treatment for this disorder and the prognosis in individual cases is largely determined by the presence and extent of neurological involvement. In the acute infantile forms, death usually occurs before the third year of life, while the chronic forms carry a better outlook, with some patients living well into adult life.

Final diagnosis

Niemann–Pick disease.

Slide 45

a. This woman has marked bruising of the lower limbs. Possible causes include:
   (i)   Trauma.
   (ii)   DIC.
   (iii) Thrombocytopenia.
b. FBC, including platelet count.
   Blood film for evidence of red cell fragmentation and DIC.
   Coagulation screen including fibrinogen and XDPs.

This woman actually had chronic ITP with demonstrable autoantibodies active against her platelets. She had been treated successfully but following an upper respiratory tract infection her platelet count had fallen from $193 \times 10^9/l$ to $2 \times 10^9/l$. This led to her marked spontaneous bruising, as shown.

> DIC would have been detected from the coagulation screen with a prolonged PT and APTT with diminished fibrinogen and increased fibrin degradation products. Microangiopathic changes would have been detected by examination of the peripheral blood film which would show red cell fragmentation.

Final diagnosis

Relapsed ITP.

Slide 46

a. The blood film consists of many atypical lymphocytes with large amounts of pale cytoplasm which appears to 'flow' around the red blood cells.
b. The commonest cause of atypical lymphocytes is infectious mononucleosis. Atypical lymphocytes are seen with other viral infections including CMV, HIV, influenza, hepatitis A and adenovirus. They are also seen in toxoplasmosis.
c. The Paul–Bunnell test detects heterophile antibodies against sheep red blood cells and is used to confirm the diagnosis of EBV infection. Peak titres are found during the second and third week of infection. Viral serology, particularly a rise in IgM antibody, is also informative.

Final diagnosis

Viral infection with atypical lymphocytes in the peripheral blood.

Slide 47

a. An abnormal neutrophil with bilobed nucleus. These are termed Pelger cells (in the familial Pelger–Huët anomaly) or pseudo-Pelger cells if they occur in myelodysplasia.
b. The most likely underlying disorder is myelodysplasia.
c. If anaemia is symptomatic, red cell transfusions may be used. For thrombocytopenia-related bleeding, regular platelet transfusions are given along with tranexamic acid. If severely neutropenic (neutrophils $<0.5 \times 10^9/l$) clinicians may use prophylactic antibacterial and antifungal agents.

Myelodysplasia is described in detail in the Review articles (Chapter 7).

Final diagnosis

Myelodysplasia; atypical Pelger neutrophils.

Slide 48

a. There is gross hypocellularity of the bone marrow with virtual absence of haematopoietic cells and replacement by fat. The bone trabeculae look normal. The appearances are those found in aplastic anaemia.
b. (i) Drugs:
   – Dose-related/predictable: cytotoxic agents.
   – Idiosyncratic: e.g. chloramphenicol, gold salts, phenylbutazone, sulphonamides, antidepressants.
   (ii) Irradiation.
   (iii) Post-viral: e.g. hepatitis A, EBV.
   (iv) Congenital: Fanconi anaemia, dyskeratosis congenita.

   Approximately two-thirds of cases of acquired aplastic anaemia are idiopathic in that no definite cause is found. An immune basis may, however, be suspected in many of the 'idiopathic' cases, as there is often a favourable response to immunosuppressive therapy (antithymocyte globulin, cyclosporin A).
   Investigation of bone marrow hypoplasia should include a Ham's acid lysis test to exclude PNH. Reduced cellularity may also be seen as a prodrome in ALL and in hypoplastic MDS.

Final diagnosis

Idiopathic aplastic anaemia.

Slide 49

a. Engorged veins.
   Retinal haemorrhages.
   Blurred optic disc.
b. The appearances are characteristic of hyperviscosity syndrome. This may result from raised levels of paraprotein in multiple myeloma or the IgM paraprotein in Waldenström's macroglobulinaemia, but also occurs in conditions with excess numbers of cells in the blood (polycythaemic states and the extreme leukocytosis which can be demonstrated with acute myelomonocytic leukaemias and the presentation of CML).

> Acute hyperviscosity syndrome will respond dramatically to plasmapheresis or cytapheresis, which need to be combined with cytotoxic therapy to reduce the underlying tumour mass and prevent rapid reaccumulation of the abnormal M-protein or cellular component. The retinal changes may improve significantly after such treatment.

The patient illustrated suffered from multiple myeloma, with an IgG paraprotein of 95 g/l at the time the photograph was obtained.

Final diagnosis

IgG myeloma with hyperviscosity.

Slide 50

a. The stain shown is a reticulin stain. This demonstrates reticulin fibres in the trephine biopsy. This specimen shows marked increase in reticulin indicating that the marrow is fibrotic. Due to the increased reticulin a dry tap is often the result of attempted marrow aspiration.
b. Any disorder causing marrow fibrosis, but the likeliest cause is myelofibrosis, one of the myeloproliferative disorders.
c. The patient will probably be anaemic and may also have abnormalities of the white cells and/or platelets. Symptomatic anaemia may require supportive blood transfusion. Thrombocytopenia causing symptoms may require platelet transfusions. Symptomatic splenomegaly may be managed by splenectomy in selected cases. In elderly patients splenic irradiation can be helpful.

Myelofibrosis is a disorder with intense fibrosis of the marrow. This may progress to thick collagen bands (especially type III collagen). The disorder has a median age of 60 years, M=F; 25% are asymptomatic at the time of diagnosis. Symptoms include weight loss, sweats, bone pain, fatigue, left upper-quadrant discomfort (spleen), hepatic enlargement. Anaemia is common with teardrop poikilocytes seen on the film. There may be an element of haemolysis and occasionally Coombs' positivity. The blood film may show nucleated red cells and myelocytes (i.e. leukoerythroblastic). The marrow aspirate is difficult to obtain (dry tap) and trephine biopsy demonstrates the features already described.

The median survival is 5 years from diagnosis and treatment is essentially supportive.

Final diagnosis

Myelofibrosis.

Slide 51

a. There are abnormal lymphocytes on the film. These are larger than normal lymphocytes and, like mature lymphocytes, have condensed chromatin. They may either represent CLL or the leukaemic phase of NHL. The red cells and platelets appear normal.
b. CLL is the likeliest diagnosis.

CLL is the commonest leukaemia in western society and affects the middle-aged/elderly. The disorder is a relatively mature clonal B cell malignancy. The aetiology is unknown; there may be hereditary factors (based on families where more than one member has the disease). Chromosomal abnormalities are common (50%). The disorder is frequently diagnosed by chance and is often asymptomatic. In other cases, the patients present with lymphadenopathy, splenomegaly, 'B' symptoms or signs of marrow failure. Immunophenotypic and other characteristics are described in the Review articles (Chapter 7).

Final diagnosis

CLL.

Slide 52

a. Gross red-cell anisopoikilocytosis, prominent target cells and sickled red cells.

The likely diagnosis is haemoglobin SC disease.

b. The patient may have aseptic necrosis of the femoral head.

> HbSC is found in compound heterozygotes who have HbS and HbC. The condition is a clinically milder sickling disorder than homozygous HbS (i.e. SS). The Hb tends to be around 11 g/dl. Growth and development are normal. The blood film, as in this case, demonstrates target cells (HbC) and sickle cells (HbS).
>
> The sickling phenomenon seen is due to polymerization of HbS and the level of HbS found in HbSC is higher than that found in sickle cell trait (where the phenotype is HbAS, i.e. HbA + HbS). Although milder than HbSS, there are certain features found in SC disease such as proliferative retinopathy that are worse than in HbSS. Aseptic necrosis of the femoral head is a feature, along with bone marrow embolism and haematuria due to renal medullary infarction.

Final diagnosis

HbSC disease.

3 | # Clinical cases

Clinical case 1

A 79-year-old man was admitted to hospital for assessment having recently deteriorated at home. He had a past history of cerebrovascular disease including left hemiparesis some weeks before admission. His family were concerned because he was falling at home and was suffering excessive bruising. On examination he was barely conscious; he had extensive bruising, both fresh and old, over his chest, abdomen and inner thighs. His temperature was normal. He was pale but well perfused. Chest examination revealed coarse crepitations. Abdominal examination was normal. Blood tests were performed on arrival at hospital, the results of which were as follows:

Hb 9.5 g/dl
MCV 95 fl
WBC $45 \times 10^9/l$
neutrophils $41.3 \times 10^9/l$

serum urea 31.8 mmol/l
serum creatinine 395 μmol/l
serum potassium 4.5 mmol/l
serum albumin 28 g/l
serum bilirubin 24 μmol/l

PT 19 s (normal range 12.0–14.0 s)
APTT 90 s (normal range 26.0–33.5 s)
fibrinogen 1.3 g/l (normal range 2.0–4.0 g/l)
XDPs >2000 μg/l (normal <250 μg/l)

a. What further investigations would you perform?
b. What is the likely diagnosis?
c. How would you manage this patient?

Clinical case 2

A 75-year-old woman was admitted under the care of the geriatricians for general assessment. She had been found to be anaemic 2 weeks previously when a domiciliary visit was carried out. Over the past 5 years she had been admitted with a variety of complaints, including mild transient ischaemic attacks, chest infections, a urinary tract infection and polymyalgia rheumatica.

Her medication consisted of bendrofluazide, digoxin, prochlorperazine, lactulose, diclofenac and prednisolone 15 mg/day. On admission various routine blood tests were carried out, the results of which were as follows:

Hb 9.6 g/dl
MCV 95 fl
WBC 5.3 × 10⁹/l
platelets 567 × 10⁹/l
ESR 58 mm/1st hour (Westergren)

serum urea 14.5 mmol/l
serum creatinine 189 μmol/l
serum potassium 4.2 mmol/l
serum calcium 2.55 mmol/l

urinalysis: trace of non-haemolysed blood; no protein detected

a. Why might this patient be anaemic?
b. What further investigations may help you confirm the diagnosis?

Clinical case 3

A 59-year-old retired office worker was admitted for investigation at his GP's request. The patient presented with a 6-week history of progressive right-sided weakness affecting the arm more than the leg. He had also developed a right-sided facial weakness. He denied any previous illnesses. His GP had checked an FBC and found mild anaemia and thrombocytopenia. His past medical history revealed appendicectomy aged 16 years but no other operations. There were no other serious illnesses of note.

He had lived and worked in North America between 1968 and 1976, after which he returned to the UK. He was single, an ex-smoker of 20 years and drank alcohol socially.

Initial investigations showed the following:

Hb 10.8 g/dl
MCV 88 fl
WBC 2.9 × 10⁹/l
neutrophils 1.0 × 10⁹/l
platelets 58 × 10⁹/l
ESR 22 mm/1st hour (Westergren)

serum B_{12} and folate – normal
serum ferritin 337 μg/l (normal range 15–300 μg/l)

serum urea 4.7 mmol/l
serum creatinine 77 μmol/l
serum potassium 3.8 mmol/l
serum calcium 2.39 mmol/l
serum albumin 37 g/l
serum gamma glutamyl transferase 26 i.u./l

a. Suggest further investigations relevant in this patient.
b. What possible diagnoses would fit these data?

Clinical case 4

A 21-year-old single trainee manageress presented to her GP with a 4-week history of increasing fatigue and general lassitude. She had been sleeping a great deal, was short of breath on minimal exertion, e.g. climbing stairs. She also commented on a feeling of 'blacking out' although she denied actual loss of consciousness. She had lost around 15–20 kg over a 3-month period. She also noticed anorexia but had no nausea, vomiting or abdominal pain. There was no overt blood loss. Her periods were regular and normal. She denied any recent foreign travel. Past medical history was unremarkable. She was taking no regular medication apart from the oral contraceptive pill, which she had been taking until 1 month before.

On examination she appeared pale but not unwell. Cardiovascular and respiratory examination was normal, as was abdominal examination. There were small nodes palpable in both axillae.

Investigations performed revealed:

Hb 5.7 g/dl
MCV 88 fl
WBC 2.3 $\times$ 10^9/l
neutrophils 1.8 $\times$ 10^9/l
platelets 100 $\times$ 10^9/l
reticulocytes 0.4%

PT 13.0 s (normal range 12.0–14.0 s)
APTT 32.0 s (normal range 26.0–33.5 s)
fibrinogen 4.3 g/l (normal range 2.0–4.0 g/l)

ESR >150 mm/1st hour (Westergren)
serum vitamin B_{12} and red cell folate-normal
serum ferritin 503 μg/l (normal range 14–200 μg/l)

serum IgG 18.1 g/l (5.3–16.5 g/l)
serum IgA 5.2 g/l (0.8–4.0 g/l)
serum IgM 1.3 g/l (0.5–2.0 g/l)

electrophoretic strip showed increased γ-globulins
C-reactive protein 11.9 mg/l (normal <6 mg/l)

a. Suggest two possible differential diagnoses.
b. What further investigations would be helpful in confirming your diagnosis?

Clinical case 5

An 85-year-old man was admitted to hospital acutely unwell. His main complaint was shortness of breath and generalized weakness. He admitted to excessive tiredness for about 4 weeks before admission and in the days prior to admission he had been unable to walk upstairs due to extreme shortness of breath. Apart from minor weight loss, he had few other systemic symptoms. He denied cough or sputum production. He had suffered no abdominal pain but did comment that he was unable to eat large amounts due to abdominal distension which he had had for several weeks before admission.

His general health had always been good and he was receiving no regular medication. His only previous admission, 10 years earlier, was for repair of an inguinal hernia.

On admission he was found to be frail but not distressed. He was clinically anaemic and appeared mildly icteric. Axillary temperature was 36.4°C. There was a small 2 cm node in the right axilla. There was no evidence of finger clubbing. Chest examination revealed occasional wheezes and abdominal examination demonstrated a fullness in the left upper quadrant with no evidence of hepatomegaly.

Investigations on arrival at hospital were:

Hb 4.7 g/dl
WBC 22.3 × 10^9/l
neutrophils 6.2 × 10^9/l
lymphocytes 15.6 × 10^9/l
MCV 130 fl
platelets 301 × 10^9/l

serum urea 9.0 mmol/l
serum creatinine 111 μmol/l
serum sodium 141 mmol/l
serum potassium 3.5 mmol/l
serum lactate dehydrogenase 1402 i.u./l

serum iron 58 μmol/l (normal range 14–33 μmol/l)
serum TIBC 48 μmol/l (normal range 45–75 μmol/l)

a. What further investigations would you request?
b. What are the differential diagnoses?

Clinical case 6

An 18-year-old student presented with a 2-day history of dull headache, fatigue and malaise. The day before she had noticed transient paraesthesiae in the left arm and apparent loss of vision for about 5 min. Two weeks earlier she had suffered from an acute febrile illness associated with nausea, vomiting and mild diarrhoea, which resolved over 3 days. Four months previously she had spent an uneventful holiday in Borneo. There was no other medical history and her only medication was the mini oral contraceptive pill.

On examination she was conscious and lucid. She was afebrile. There was marked pallor and a tinge of jaundice. A few petechiae were noted over the shins and ankles. There were no other abnormal clinical findings and in particular neurological examination was unremarkable.

Initial investigations performed were as follows:

Hb 6.2 g/dl
MCV 84 fl
WBC $17.5 \times 10^9/l$
neutrophils $12.0 \times 10^9/l$
platelets $15 \times 10^9/l$

serum urea 11.3 mmol/l
serum creatinine 126 μmol/l
serum sodium 138 mmol/l
serum potassium 4.6 mmol/l

CXR – normal

Three hours after admission the patient suddenly became confused and disorientated. On examination she was febrile (38.6°C). There were signs of cerebral irritation with brisk reflexes, but there was no neck stiffness and no focal neurological signs.

a. What urgent investigations are indicated?
b. What are the differential diagnoses?

Clinical case 7

Jane, a 32-year-mother of two children, was seen at her regular rheumatology outpatient visit. She was diagnosed as suffering from RA 8 years previously and, although not severe, radiology had shown erosive changes in the right ulnar styloid and several other joints. She was started initially on diclofenac and sulphasalazine which had been controlling the disease. More recently she had been suffering with intermittent back pain radiating down both legs, classified by the rheumatologist as the LHermitte's phenomenon. He considered the possibility of a demyelinating process, although there were few symptoms or signs to suggest this as a likely diagnosis. She gave no history suggestive of retrobulbar neuritis. She was referred for neurological investigation, and in particular evoked potentials, after suffering sensory symptoms in her left leg ('dead leg') coincident with numbness in the face. On examination at that time she demonstrated sensory loss on the left side of her face with absent corneal reflex. Limb reflexes were brisk but the left plantar response was equivocal. Visual evoked potentials were normal. These were repeated 6 months later and were clearly abnormal the report stating '... suggestive of multiple sclerosis'.

The rheumatologist arranged various blood tests, the results of which were unexpected. It was decided to seek haematological advice at this point. The results of these blood tests are shown below:

Hb 11.9 g/dl
MCV 83 fl
WBC 7.4×10^9/l
neutrophils 4.1×10^9/l
reticulocytes 1.3%

PT 14.0 s (normal range 12.0–14.0 s)
APTT 31.5 s (26.0–33.5 s)
fibrinogen 6.3 g/l (normal range 2.0–4.0 g/l)
ESR 23 mm/1st hour (Westergren)

serum IgG 35 g/l (normal range 5.3–16.5 g/l)
serum IgA 3.2 g/l (normal range 0.8–4.0 g/l)
serum IgM 1.1 g/l (normal range 0.5–2.0 g/l)

Urea and electrolytes, liver and thyroid function – normal

a. Do the patient's diagnoses account for the laboratory findings?
b. What further investigations are required in order to manage this
   patient effectively?
c. What would be your plan of action in this case?

Clinical case 8

A 17-year-old girl was seen by her GP because she had been generally unwell for about 3 months. Initially, she felt as though she had
flu with joint pains and fever but, rather than subside over a week
or so, her symptoms persisted. She noticed small glands in the neck
area and admitted to losing a few kilograms in weight over this
period. She also complained of generalized itching for the 4 weeks
before the visit to her GP.

   Her past medical history was unremarkable apart from childhood eczema and she was receiving no regular medication.
Systems review was unhelpful.

   When the GP examined her, he noted that she appeared quite
well. She was not clinically anaemic or jaundiced. She had a few
palpable lymph nodes in the cervical area, the largest of which was
3 × 3 cm in size. She had a few shotty glands in both groins but no
other palpable lymphadenopathy.

   The GP arranged for her to be seen in the haematology clinic
urgently. Initial investigations performed in clinic showed:

Hb 11.3 g/dl
MCV 84.2 fl
WBC 12.5 × 10⁹/l
neutrophils 8.1 × 10⁹/l
eosinophils 0.5 × 10⁹/l
platelets 500 × 10⁹/l
ESR 60 mm/1st hour (Westergren)

urea and electrolytes – normal
serum calcium 2.59 mmol/l
serum LDH 950 i.u./l
serum albumin 34 g/l
serum bilirubin 9 μmol/l

abdominal ultrasound: normal; no evidence of intra-abdominal lymphadenopathy

a. What is your differential diagnosis?
b. What further investigations would you arrange?

Clinical case 9

A 50-year-old shopkeeper was admitted as an emergency under the care of the general physicians with severe pneumonia. He had felt unwell for several days with cough and fever but it was only after he collapsed at work that his wife called the family doctor, who arranged the admission. He was commenced on i.v. antibiotics and oxygen and made a prompt recovery. During the admission a variety of blood tests were arranged and, in view of the results of these, radiological investigations were organized. The patient also had a bone marrow aspirate and trephine biopsy performed.

Hb 12.3 g/dl
WBC 1.8×10^9/l
neutrophils 0.6×10^9/l
eosinophils 0.02×10^9/l
atypical cells 0.14×10^9/l
platelets 60×10^9/l

urea and electrolytes – normal

abdominal ultrasound: modest enlargement of the liver suggestive of fatty infiltration. The spleen is slightly enlarged (14 cm). No evidence of lymphadenopathy

Cell markers (marrow)

CD23	0%
λ	1%
κ	23%
CD19	19%
IgG	8%
IgM	18%
IgA	1%
IgD	1%
CD22	14%
CD37	21%
CD5	2%
CD10	2%
HC2	9%
TRAP	9%

a. What are the differential diagnoses?
b. What investigation results would you review as a matter or urgency?
c. What treatment options are available?
d. What would you tell the patient about the prognosis?

Clinical case 10

A 47-year-old man was admitted to the neurology unit with severe headache and associated numbness in the left arm with tingling and occasional jerking which had occurred intermittently for the 3 weeks before admission. His past medical history was unremarkable. He was currently taking phenobarbitone 30 mg t.d.s. On examination the positive findings were of splenomegaly (2 cm) and small lymph nodes in the left supraclavicular area. It was felt that lymphoma should be excluded and a bone marrow was performed. This showed megakaryocytic hyperplasia but no evidence of lymphoma. At that time his Hb, WBC and platelets were normal. A blood film showed occasional large platelets only. Biochemistry screen was normal apart from elevated serum urate (0.6 mmol/l). Lymphangiography revealed filling defects in the superficial femoral and external iliac nodes on the left side. The right iliac nodes were reported to be 'foamy and expanded' and the para-aortic chain was deviated to the right of L2 and L3.

He was lost to follow-up and was not seen until 15 years later when he was found to have a Hb of 10.2 g/dl; WBC and platelets again were marginally reduced (3.2 and $103 \times 10^9/l$ respectively). Blood film showed leukoerythroblastic changes. Bone marrow was repeated and this showed a hypercellular marrow with increased granulocytes, megakaryocytes and reticulin fibres. Cytogenetic analysis was normal. At this point the patient complained of cough and dyspnoea. He had required several courses of antibiotics during the previous months. He had suffered severe sweats and had lost 11 kg over the past year. On examination his spleen was further enlarged with 14 cm palpable below the left costal margin. Five years later he was even more cachectic with a 24-cm spleen but no evidence of cytopenia. The leukoerythroblastic features noted earlier were still present.

a. What differential diagnoses are suggested by this clinical picture?
b. Outline the natural history of the likeliest diagnosis.

Clinical case 11

A 63-year-old female presented with persisting generalized backache and hip pain worsening over the previous 2 months. Twelve months previously she had seen her GP with an acute onset of mid-thoracic backache. Simple investigation at that time had shown osteoporosis of the spine and a wedge fracture of T12. CXR was normal. FBC taken at the time had been reported as normal and no abnormality was found on screening urea, electrolytes and calcium. She had been diagnosed as suffering post-menopausal osteoporosis and managed with simple analgesics. An attempt had been made to give calcium supplements but she had electively stopped taking these after some 6 weeks.

On presentation she complained of generalized backache, especially troublesome in the morning, and some pain and stiffness in her left hip on moving around. Her appetite was unchanged but she had lost 3 kg in the last 6 weeks. The pains were generally eased by taking co-proxamol, 2 tablets 6-hourly. She had been on no other prescribed medication but had been taking oil of evening primrose and a vitamin B complex preparation. Her past medical history was unremarkable with no previous operations; she was para 2+0. She had previously been very fit, having been a ballet dancer until her early 40s. Physical examination showed her to be of small stature with some tenderness over T10. There were no other focal abnormalities. There was no lymphadenopathy; examination of her chest revealed no abnormality; heart sounds were normal and hepatosplenomegaly was not detected.

Hb 11.8 g/dl
MCV 91 fl
WBC $5.3 \times 10^9/l$
differential WBC was normal
platelets $185 \times 10^9/l$
ESR 8 mm/1st hour (Westergren)

serum sodium 141 mmol/l
serum potassium 4.1 mmol/l
serum chloride 100 mmol/l
serum urea 5.3 mmol/l
serum creatinine 91 μmol/l
serum calcium 2.31 mmol/l
serum phosphate 1.2 mmol/l
serum total protein 68 g/l
serum albumin 31 g/l

a. Suggest two likely diagnoses.
b. List five appropriate further investigations.

Clinical case 12

A 41-year-old female complained of intermittent backache over a 4-month period. Radiology of the lumbar spine organized by her GP had been unremarkable and she referred herself to a chiropractor for manipulation. This had been carried out a month before presentation. She had noticed marked bruising over her ribs afterwards. She also felt more fatigued and developed a symptomatic respiratory infection with a cough and purulent sputum. This was treated by her GP with a 5-day course of antibiotics and seemed to resolve. She continued to complain of tiredness. FBC was checked with the following results: Hb 9.9 g/dl, MCV 93 fl, WBC $2.2 \times 10^9/l$ and platelets $97 \times 10^9/l$.

Her GP initiated referral to outpatients for further assessment. In the meantime her condition deteriorated; she complained of increased fatigue and noticed ease of bruising. Bruising was generalized and mostly not associated with known trauma. Past medical history was unremarkable. She was para1+0 and worked as a part-time sales assistant in a shoe shop until symptoms from her backache had caused her to give up this job. She had been taking co-dydramol and diclofenac fairly regularly because of persisting backache. She was a non-smoker and her alcohol consumption was

3–4 units per week. Her GP noted the increased bruising and worsening symptoms. He rechecked the blood count and the results were as follows:

Hb 8.1 g/dl
MCV 91 fl
WBC 2.4 × 10⁹/l
neutrophils 1.3 × 10⁹/l.
platelets 19 × 10⁹/l

blood film: neutropenia and circulating myelocytes with occasional nucleated red cells and teardrop poikilocytes.

Apart from bruising, the GP found nothing else on physical examination and referred her urgently for admission and further assessment. Clinical examination on admission showed the presence of generalized bruising. There was oozing from venepuncture sites and some gum bleeding. Testing also indicated the presence of microscopic haematuria. BP was 140/90 mmHg, pulse 88 beats/min and regular and temperature 37.1°C.

a. What is the likely diagnosis?
b. List five appropriate further investigations.
c. Outline the principles of initial management.

Clinical case 13

A 46-year-old Caucasian female presented to her GP with general lethargy. There were no specific findings; he checked an FBC. This showed her to be anaemic with Hb 8.6 g/dl, MCV 68 fl, total WBC 7.2 × 10⁹/l and platelets 375 × 10⁹/l. The film was reported as showing hypochromia; white cells and platelets were normal.

Brief enquiry from the GP revealed no suggested cause for iron deficiency other than menstruation. She was given ferrous sulphate 200 mg t.d.s. Her dosage had to be reduced to 200 mg daily because of side-effects of abdominal discomfort and nausea. A repeat blood count a month later showed her Hb to be 9.3 g/dl and MCV 70 fl. The GP had organized a serum ferritin estimation after her initial blood count; iron deficiency was confirmed by finding a low ferritin of 1 μg/l (normal 14–200 μg/l). Her symptoms and signs were reviewed but no clear cause was found for her persisting anaemia and she was referred for further assessment. On referral she was well but continued to complain of ease of fatigue.

Her weight had been steady and her appetite reasonable. She was a housewife with a part-time job. She cooked for herself, her two teenage children and husband. Her diet appeared to be normal and she was on no regular medication. She took paracetamol occasionally for dysmenorrhoeic symptoms. She had been a blood donor and her last donation was 5 years previously. Her menstrual cycle was 6 days every 28 days; periods were described as 'quite heavy' but had not changed recently. Clinical examination was unremarkable; there was no lymphadenopathy. Temperature, pulse and BP were all normal. Examination of her chest revealed no abnormality. Abdominal examination was unremarkable apart from some non-specific periumbilical tenderness.

Hb 9.3 g/dl
MCV 70 fl
WBC 6.8×10^9/l
platelets 393×10^9/l
ESR 21 mm/1st hour (Westergren)

serum urea and electrolytes – normal
serum calcium 2.23 mmol/l
serum alanine aminotransferase 33 i.u./l (normal 5–42 i.u./l)
serum ferritin 3 μg/l (normal range 14–200 μg/l)
serum vitamin B_{12} 195 ng/l (normal 150–700 ng/l)
serum and red cell folate – normal

Because of side-effects associated with oral iron supplementation, she received an i.v. infusion of iron dextran. FBC 3 weeks later showed Hb 12.2 g/dl, MCV 85 fl, total WBC 5.9×10^9/l and platelets 390×10^9/l. Three months later she returned with a recurrence of previous symptoms. Hb was 9.8 g/dl, MCV 71 fl, total WBC 8.1×10^9/l, platelets 401×10^9/l.

a. What is the likely reason for her anaemia?
b. Suggest five helpful further investigations.

Clinical case 14

A 26-year-old man sustained a large haematoma over his right hip following a minor fall. This was investigated with an FBC which showed Hb 12.0 g/dl, MCV 88 fl, WBC 7.1 × 10^9/l and platelets 61 × 10^9/l.

He was referred for evaluation. He had previously been well; there was nothing of note in his past medical history. He had been involved in a road traffic accident 4 years previously and had marked bruising associated with seat belt injuries which resolved uneventfully. He had been on no recent medication; he worked as a civil servant, and was married with one child aged 3 years. Clinical examination showed a resolving haematoma over the hip. There were no other general abnormalities of note. Lymphadenopathy was not present; clinical hepatosplenomegaly was noted. The liver edge was palpable 3 cm below the costal margin; the spleen tip could be palpated 10 cm below the costal margin. Both were smooth and non-tender.

Hb 13.0 g/dl
MCV 82 fl
WBC 4.6 × 10^9/l with a normal differential count
platelets 62 × 10^9/l

PT 16 s (normal range 12.0–14.0 s)
APTT 65 s (normal range 26.0–33.5 s)
fibrinogen 1.7 g/l (normal range 2.0–4.0 g/l)

serum sodium 139 mmol/l
serum potassium 3.5 mmol/l
serum bicarbonate 27 mmol/l
serum urea 4.5 mmol/l
serum creatinine 84 μmol/l
serum calcium 2.25 mmol/l
serum phosphate 1.26 mmol/l
serum total protein 72 g/l
serum albumin 44 g/l
serum bilirubin 14 μmol/l
serum alkaline phosphatase 112 i.u./l
serum alanine aminotransferase 34 i.u./l

a. What seems the likely diagnosis?
b. What further diagnostic tests would you arrange?
c. Suggest appropriate further management.

Clinical case 15

A 66-year-old housewife was referred by a rheumatologist for haematological review. She had suffered with mild RA for 10 years. The disease affected the small joints of her hands predominantly and currently the condition was quiescent. She had been feeling particularly depressed and was having problems at home with her husband who suffered with senile dementia. In the past 3 months before being reviewed she had suffered two chest infections which each took 3 weeks or more to resolve completely, despite adequate antibiotic therapy. Currently she was quite well and was taking occasional diclofenac for joint pains. She was also taking isosorbide mononitrate and bendrofluazide regularly for hypertension. It had been noted that two recent FBCs had demonstrated a reduction in the neutrophil and platelet counts; her Hb was mildly reduced.

On examination she appeared anxious and slightly tearful. She was not clinically anaemic or jaundiced and there were no palpable lymph nodes. Examination of the cardiovascular, respiratory and GI systems was normal; in particular she had no palpable spleen. The rheumatologist rechecked her FBC and biochemistry screen:

Hb 10.4 g/dl
WBC 2.3 × 10^9/l
neutrophils 0.4 × 10^9/l
platelets 75 × 10^9/l
ESR 24 mm/1st hour (Westergren)

urea, electrolytes and liver function tests – normal

peripheral blood cell markers:

Monoclonal Antibody	% positive cells
CD34	1%
HLA class II	40%
κ	8%
λ	5%
CD8	63%
CD4	27%
CD19	8%
CD3	88%

a. Suggest two causes for the abnormal blood findings.
b. List four investigations which may help you reach a diagnosis.
c. Outline your management of this patient.

Clinical case 16

A 59-year-old man presented with weakness and weight loss of 17 kg over the preceding 6 months. He had also noticed joint pains affecting particularly the small joints of his right hand and his knees. He had been diagnosed as suffering from diabetes mellitus 5 years previously and was managed by diet and oral hypoglycaemic agents. He was on no other medication. In the family history, his brother had died of malignant disease at the age of 62 years and he had a sister who was alive and well. He smoked 15 cigarettes each day and drank beer and spirits on a regular basis.

Examination revealed a thin man with palmar erythema and mild bilateral Dupuytren's contractures. There was a small area of increased pigmentation of the skin over the back of the left hand. There was no clinical jaundice but three spider naevi were present over the upper trunk. The liver was enlarged 7 cm below the right costal margin and the spleen was tippable. There was no ascites.

Initial investigations were as follows:

Hb 15.1 g/dl
MCV 102 fl
WBC 10.1 × 10^9/l
platelets 215 × 10^9/l

serum sodium 141 mmol/l
serum potassium 4.5 mmol/l
serum urea 6.0 mmol/l
serum creatinine 96 μmol/l
serum bilirubin 15 μmol/l
serum alkaline phosphatase 125 i.u./l
serum alanine aminotransferase 105 i.u./l
serum gamma glutamyl transferase 117 i.u./l
fasting glucose 17 mmol/l

serum vitamin B_{12} 780 ng/l (normal 150–700 ng/l)
red cell folate 175 μg/l (normal 150–700 μg/l)
serum ferritin 1205 μg/l (normal range 15–300 μg/l)

a. What is the differential diagnosis apart from his diabetes?
b. What further investigations are indicated?

Clinical case 17

A 73-year-old woman with unexplained anaemia, was referred for haematology opinion. She had suffered a chest infection 1 year before which was treated with erythromycin. She had been taking regular captopril for hypertension for the past 5 years. She was symptomatically well, denied any overt blood loss, had a good appetite and her weight was steady. She had recently undergone dental extraction which was complicated by 'reactionary haemorrhage' requiring packing. On examination she seemed well, although was clinically anaemic. There was no evidence of jaundice and she had no palpable glands. A bone marrow was performed by a local haematologist and this appeared normal. Investigation at that time showed:

Hb 9.4 g/dl
MCV 82 fl
WBC $3.5 \times 10^9/l$
neutrophils $2.2 \times 10^9/l$
lymphocytes $1.2 \times 10^9/l$
platelets $135 \times 10^9/l$
ESR 18 mm/1st hour (Westergren)

serum urea 5.3 mmol/l
serum creatinine 89 μmol/l
serum calcium 2.33 mmol/l
serum sodium 141 mmol/l
serum potassium 4.4 mmol/l
serum bilirubin 7 μmol/l
serum alkaline phosphatase 115 i.u./l
serum total protein 81 g/l

After haematological review a second marrow was performed along with repeat FBC which showed:

Hb 7.4 g/dl
MCV 86.5 fl
WBC $9.0 \times 10^9/l$
neutrophils $6.0 \times 10^9/l$
platelets $55 \times 10^9/l$

Marrow aspirate showed hypercellularity with dysplastic changes noted in all three cell lines.

Marrow trephine confirmed hypercellularity with increased reticulin and an increase in intermediate-stage myeloid cells.

serum B_{12} 1427 ng/l (normal 150–700 ng/l)
red cell folate 513 μg/l (normal 150–700 μg/l)
ferritin 80 μg/l (normal range 15–300 μg/l)

a. What do you feel is the likeliest diagnosis?
b. What treatment options are available?
c. What is the prognosis in this condition?

Clinical case 18

An anxious 30-year-old mother of one young girl sought an appointment with her family doctor because of exhaustion. She complained of recurrent epistaxes every 10 days lasting about 10 min each time. These had been occurring for about 4 months in total. In addition, she had noticed bruising over her lower extremities, especially at the top of her thighs.

She was in good general health but had suffered a recent bout of depression leading to her being given Prozac, which she felt had started the whole chain of events. Her diet was good and her weight steady. She denied any genitourinary or GI upset. Her periods were regular but tended to last for 7 days and were fairly heavy.

Her past medical history consisted of pyeloplasty 20 years previously and a caesarean section 3 years before. She had also suffered miscarriages 5 and 4 years earlier.

On examination she was pale but not jaundiced. She had a small posterior auricular lymph node on the right side. She also had a small axillary node on the left side. Breast examination was normal, as was examination of respiratory, cardiovascular systems and abdomen.

The GP was unsure what these symptoms and signs amounted to but performed a FBC which showed:

Hb 7.9 g/dl
MCV 71.3 fl
WBC 4.5 × 10^9/l
neutrophils 2.1 × 10^9/l
platelets 256 × 10^9/l

a. From the available results are there any further investigations you would like to perform?
b. What do these indices suggest to you?
c. What treatment would you recommend?

Clinical case 19

A 37-year-old man was admitted with lassitude, dyspnoea, pyrexia, a non-productive cough and left-sided variable chest pain over the previous 2–3 days; his symptoms were not improving despite 48 h of oral amoxycillin prescribed by his family doctor. He had been on no regular medication and had consulted the practice very occasionally beforehand. He had been off his work, as an electrician, 3 months previously for an episode of jaundice which had fully settled.

On admission he was noted to be unwell and pale with a temperature of 38.9°C; pulse 110 beats/min and regular; BP 110/70 mmHg. There were two small mouth ulcers. Examination of his chest revealed left-sided crepitations and a pleural rub. Abdominal examination was normal. CXR showed shadowing at the left base. Blood cultures were taken and he was commenced on empirical i.v. antibiotic therapy. Other results are shown below:

Hb 5.9 g/dl
MCV 101 fl
WBC $0.8 \times 10^9/l$
Neutrophils $0.1 \times 10^9/l$
Platelets $10 \times 10^9/l$

serum urea 9.1 mmol/l
serum creatinine 96 μmol/l

Blood cultures: no growth

a. Suggest two likely diagnoses.
b. Indicate three further tests likely to be of diagnostic value.
c. Outline your immediate management of the problem.

Clinical case 20

A 22-year-old trainee manageress was referred for further investigation. She gave a history of generalized lassitude and recurrent sore throats since an episode of 'glandular fever' some 18 months previously. She had to take time off during periods of fatigue and she also complained of occasional episodes of feeling hot. At the time of her glandular fever illness she had lymphadenopathy which subsequently regressed. During the periods of fatigue she felt that her submandibular and cervical lymph nodes became enlarged. She was para 0+0 with no other significant past medical history. She smoked about 5 cigarettes a day and her alcohol intake was around 3 units per week. Her periods were regular and not heavy. She lived with her fiancé and, until 6 months previously, had been taking the oral contraceptive pill.

On clinical examination her temperature was 37.2°C, pulse 68 beats/min and regular, BP 120/80 mmHg. There was 2–3 cm non-tender enlargement of cervical, submandibular, axillary and iliac nodes. There was no hepatosplenomegaly. In the referral letter from her GP blood tests at the time of her viral infection had been unremarkable. A blood count at the time of referral showed:

Hb 11.7 g/dl
MCV 89 fl
WBC $3.7 \times 10^9/l$
neutrophils $1.9 \times 10^9/l$
platelets $83 \times 10^9/l$
ESR 72 mm/1st hour (Westergren)

peripheral blood film: unremarkable

coagulation screen: normal with no evidence for the lupus anticoagulant
autoimmune profile: negative
CXR: normal

Results of the urea, electrolytes and liver function tests are listed:

serum sodium 139 mmol/l
serum potassium 3.9 mmol/l
serum bicarbonate 27 mmol/l
serum chloride 100 mmol/l
serum urea 5.1 mmol/l
serum creatinine 83 μmol/l
serum calcium 2.31 mmol/l
serum albumin 30 g/l
serum alkaline phosphatase 220 i.u./l
serum aspartate transaminase 38 i.u./l

a. Specify three investigations likely to be clinically helpful.
b. Indicate three possible differential diagnoses.

Clinical case 21

A 71-year-old female presented with a 3-week history of being generally unwell. Predominant symptoms included joint pains and general malaise. The joints mostly affected were hands, wrists and knees. Symptoms were partially relieved by paracetamol or ibuprofen obtained through the local pharmacy. She complained of intermittent fevers and had eventually consulted her GP after a week of anorexia accompanied by night sweats.

Further information from her GP indicated a history of exertional dyspnoea and generalized leg pains over the same period of time.

Her past medical history was unremarkable. She was retired, single and lived with her brother and another friend in a bungalow. Three years previously she had had an episode of herpes zoster which settled without complication. She formerly smoked up to 30 cigarettes a day but had given up at the time of the zoster episode.

Clinical examination was unremarkable. There was mild tenderness in the proximal interphalangeal and metacarpophalangeal joints of both hands. She was pale and dyspnoeic on modest effort. Pulse was 72 beats/min and regular. BP was 120/80 mmHg. Temperature was 37.5°C. There was no lymphadenopathy. An apical systolic murmur with radiation to the axilla was noted. She was obese but there was no clinical hepatosplenomegaly.

Investigations showed:

Hb 8.1 g/dl
MCV 92 fl
WBC $1.7 \times 10^9/l$
neutrophils $0.1 \times 10^9/l$
platelets $244 \times 10^9/l$

ESR 130 mm/1st hour (Westergren)

a. What is the likely diagnosis in this case?
b. Suggest three further appropriate investigations.

Clinical case 22

A 75-year-old woman was admitted under the elderly care physicians for assessment following a visit by her GP. She had been non-specifically unwell for a number of weeks but had become significantly worse with nausea, anorexia and mild weight loss. During the hospital admission a variety of blood tests and other investigations were performed:

Hb 9.3 g/dl
RCC 3.5×10^{12}/l
MCV 82 fl
MCH 26.6 pg
MCHC 32.6 g/dl
PCV 0.285
WBC 14.3×10^9/l
neutrophils 10×10^9/l
ESR 34 mm/1st hour (Westergren)

serum vitamin B_{12} 818 ng/l (normal 150–700 ng/l)
serum ferritin 38 μg/l (normal range 15–300 μg/l)
red cell folate 756 μg/l (normal 150–700 μg/l)

PT 13.0 s (control 12.0–14.0 s)
APTT 29.3 s (control 26.0–33.5 s)
serum sodium 137 mmol/l
serum potassium 4.7 mmol/l
serum urea 15.2 mmol/l
serum creatinine 135 μmol/l
serum calcium 2.23 mmol/l
serum albumin 16 g/l
serum total bilirubin 89 μmol/l
serum alkaline phosphatase 1445 i.u./l
serum alanine aminotransferase 44 i.u./l
serum gamma glutamyl transferase 69 i.u./l
random blood glucose 6.0 mmol/l
free T_4 10.4 pmol/l (normal range 9–24 pmol/l)
TSH 17.1 mU/l (normal range 0.35–5.5 mU/l)

a. What aspects of the patient's history would you like to know?
b. What further tests would you arrange?
c. Suggest three possible diagnoses.

Clinical case 23

A 63-year-old retired surveyor presented to his GP complaining of increasing fatigue and a mild degree of exertional dyspnoea. He had previously been fit and a BUPA medical 18 months previously had shown him to be in normal health apart from a modest elevation of blood pressure, for which his GP had treated him with a small dose of a beta-blocker. Nothing else of note was found by the GP on presentation.

A blood count was organized and this showed:

Hb 8.5 g/dl
MCV 65 fl
WBC 8.3 × 10^9/l
platelets 443 × 10^9/l

ESR 43 mm/1st hour (Westergren)

Hypochromic changes were noticed in the blood film; white cell appearances were unremarkable.

The GP checked serum iron and iron-binding capacity and started him on iron supplements. Serum iron was 5 μmol/l (normal range 14–33 μmol/l), total iron-binding capacity was 51 μmol/l (normal range 45–75 μmol/l). The patient was referred directly for a gastroscopy and a barium enema. Gastroscopy showed a small hiatus hernia and was otherwise entirely normal. Barium enema was a satisfactory examination with no abnormality found apart from occasional diverticula. Faecal occult bloods were checked; two were negative, one was positive.

An FBC check 1 month after starting iron supplements and a further 6 weeks later showed no change in the values. He was referred for further assessment at that time:

Hb 9.1 g/dl
MCV 69 fl
WBC 9.1 × 10^9/l
platelets 444 × 10^9/l
ESR 51 mm/1st hour (Westergren)

a. Suggest two alternative causes for this anaemia.
b. List four investigations that might be of further diagnostic help.

Clinical case 24

A 75-year-old Caucasian male presented with lassitude, 5 kg weight loss and variable night sweats. His symptoms were of 4 months' duration; previous to this he had been in good health. He retired at 65 from work in a cable manufacturing plant. In retirement he had remained active, playing percussion in a local dance band, gardening and golfing. These activities had reduced in the last 3 months. He described some dyspnoea walking up hills in cold weather and experienced occasional heartburn. There was sensation of occasional muscle discomfort and stiffness in his shoulders. He had been a non-smoker for over 40 years. Alcohol intake was minimal.

His GP had found nothing on initial assessment. A blood count was taken and indicated the following results: Hb 10.5 g/dl, MCV 77 fl, WBC 27.2 × 10^9/l, platelets 375 × 10^9/l, ESR 38 mm in the first hour. Blood film: neutrophilia, occasional myelocytes. Physical examination on referral was unremarkable apart from 4 cm of non-tender hepatomegaly and 6 cm of non-tender splenomegaly. He was admitted for further investigation and observation because of persisting symptoms and anxiety about the symptoms. The results of investigations performed on admission showed:

Hb 10.7 g/dl
MCV 77 fl
WBC 34.3 × 10^9/l
platelets 377 × 10^9/l
ESR 53 mm/1st hour (Westergren)

Blood film: neutrophilia, myelocytes, metamyelocytes, occasional blast cells, teardrop poikilocytes, occasional nucleated red cells

serum ferritin 377 μg/l (normal range 15–300 μg/l)

serum sodium 139 mmol/l
serum potassium 3.9 mmol/l
serum chloride 101 mmol/l
serum bicarbonate 27 mmol/l
serum urea 7.0 mmol/l
serum creatinine 110 μmol/l
serum total protein 72 g/l
serum albumin 36 g/l
serum bilirubin 20 μmol/l
serum alkaline phosphatase 813 i.u./l
serum aspartate transaminase 53 i.u./l

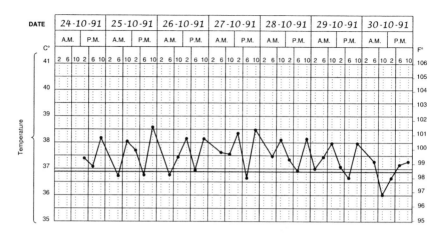

Fig. 3.1 Patient's temperature chart over 7-day period showing fluctuating pyrexia.

CXR: non-specific shadowing at left costophrenic angle. Otherwise normal

Abdominal and pelvic ultrasound: no lymphadenopathy seen

A fluctuating pyrexia was noted (Fig. 3.1)

Bone marrow aspirate and biopsy were undertaken.
Aspirate: cellular with all lines increased.
Trephine biopsy: showed maximal cellularity with some irregularity of megakaryocyte distribution. The features were consistent with cellular-phase myelofibrosis.

It was concluded that his symptoms were due to myelofibrosis. He was given hydroxyurea which reduced the total WBC to the normal range but produced no change in symptoms. Because of persisting symptoms and a transfusion dependency it was decided to perform splenectomy. Preoperative Pneumovax was given; splenectomy was carried out 10 days later and was uneventful. He was given long-term oral penicillin.

Three weeks afterwards he was admitted with profound lethargy and fever. He had lost a further 5 kg in weight; there was a cough with purulent sputum. He was treated with i.v. antibiotics, and the temperature did improve. He remained generally lethargic. He was commenced on prednisolone 25 mg daily tailing by 5 mg each week as a non-specific symptomatic treatment for myelofibrosis.

There was a distinct symptomatic benefit. Four weeks later Hb was 8.4 g/dl and he was admitted for a supportive transfusion. Prednisolone dosage was 5 mg daily and he had started to experience lassitude. Clinical assessment demonstrated the presence of right-sided supraclavicular lymphadenopathy.

a. What is your differential diagnosis?
b. Suggest four immediately helpful investigations.

Clinical case 25

A 23-year-old man presented with generalized fatigue and intermittent backache. His symptoms had started some 6 months previously following a short flu-like illness. Since then he had described recurrent sore throats lasting 1–2 days and a variable degree of fatigue. He had taken time off his work in the local tax office on some three occasions during that time. His initial illness was treated with an antibiotic from his GP. With the antibiotic he developed a rash. A blood count was performed and he was advised that a test for glandular fever had proved positive.

On further enquiry he had lost some 4 kg in weight a month after his initial illness. Over the next 3 months he lost a further 2 kg but he had regained this in the month prior to presentation. There was little else of note in his past medical history; he had had an ear infection with grommet insertion as a child. Because of irregular bowel habit and intermittent diarrhoea he had been investigated at a gastroenterology clinic 2 years previously and diagnosed as having irritable bowel.

The family history revealed that his mother had been diagnosed 12 months previously as having breast cancer; the lump was removed and she had completed 6 months of chemotherapy. His father was well, and he had two siblings who were well. One cousin had died some 8 years previously from leukaemia. He lived locally with his parents; he was a non-smoker. His alcohol intake was estimated at 14–21 units per week.

The GP referred him because of persisting symptoms. In the referral letter the GP indicated that a leukocytosis with atypical lymphocytes was recorded during the initial illness. Follow-up blood counts had shown resolution of the lymphocytosis but he had continued to run a neutropenia of between 1.2 and 1.6 × 10⁹/l on two subsequent blood counts.

The history and findings were confirmed on initial referral. There was no particular pattern to his symptoms. His fatigue had worsened in the previous month and he also described a variable degree of aching in his back. He also described some pain and discomfort in his legs which had woken him during the night, for which he had needed to take paracetamol. He had no other medication. Physical examination showed pallor, pulse was 68 beats/min and regular, blood pressure 110/70 mmHg. His chest was clear, heart sounds were normal and abdominal examination was unremarkable.

FBC showed:

Hb 12.7 g/dl
MCV 92 fl
WBC 3.2 × 10^9/l
platelets 143 × 10^9/l
neutrophils 0.9 × 10^9/l
ESR 29 mm/1st hour (Westergren)

Glandular fever screening test (Monospot) – negative

Blood film: occasional atypical lymphoid cell noted

serum sodium 138 mmol/l
serum potassium 4.1 mmol/l
serum bicarbonate 26 mmol/l
serum chloride 101 mmol/l
serum urea 5.2 mmol/l
serum creatinine 89 μmol/l
serum total protein 78 g/l
serum albumin 39 g/l
serum bilirubin 19 μmol/l
serum alkaline phosphatase 410 i.u./l
serum aspartate transaminase 39 i.u./l

a. List four possible differential diagnoses.
b. Recommend four helpful investigations.

Answers to clinical cases

Clinical case 1

a. Platelet count.
   Peripheral blood film examination.
   Blood cultures.
   CXR.
   Urinalysis and culture of MSU.
   CT brain scan.
b. Based on the clinical findings and the results provided, this man appears to have DIC. He has suffered unexplained bruising and appears to have had a recent cerebrovascular event. From the FBC provided he has a significant neutrophilia and normocytic anaemia. The coagulation tests are highly suggestive of DIC since both PT and APTT are prolonged and the XDPs (released after the formation of fibrin) are grossly elevated. Furthermore, the fibrinogen is below the normal level – a feature characteristic of DIC. Since platelets are consumed in the DIC process the platelet count tends to be low. This was not provided with the initial FBC and should be requested urgently.

DIC may occur in a variety of settings, including infection, hence the need to perform blood and urine cultures. If sputum is being expectorated this, too, should be sent for culture and sensitivity. Other causes of DIC are: malignancy, including acute leukaemias (especially APML), obstetric emergencies (amniotic fluid embolism, eclampsia), hypersensitivity reactions, incompatible blood transfusions, liver failure, severe burns, massive tissue injury, carcinoma, snake bites, anaphylaxis, etc.

DIC results in widespread deposition of fibrin in small blood vessels that causes tissue and organ damage through ischaemia. Because clotting factors are depleted, the patient suffers bleeding complications. DIC is estimated to occur in 1 : 1000 hospital admissions.

In acute DIC the PT and APTT are prolonged, the platelets are reduced and the XDPs are elevated. In chronic DIC, however, the clotting factors and platelets may be normal but XDPs are elevated and there will be red cell fragments on the blood film.

c.   The management of DIC remains controversial: the most important aspect consists of treating of the underlying cause. If this is achieved, then the DIC often resolves fairly rapidly. However, patients often require intensive supportive care and this is provided by blood transfusion, together with administration of fresh frozen plasma and cryoprecipitate to replace clotting factors consumed in the DIC process.

Platelets may be given if life-threatening bleeding is likely or evident. One school of thought believes that administration of blood components may add to the DIC by providing exogenous clotting factors. However, most clinicians would advocate their use if the patient is actively bleeding.

Some haematologists advocate the use of i.v. heparin but there is no overall consensus of opinion on the role of anticoagulation in DIC. Theoretically heparin should help since heparin activates antithrombin III which neutralizes free thrombin and further inhibits its formation. Heparin may be useful when thrombosis is clinically evident. No randomized trials to date have shown any benefit in terms of outcome of patients who have received heparin in the setting of DIC.

Final diagnosis

DIC secondary to underlying prostatic carcinoma.

Clinical case 2

a. Underlying renal impairment.
   Non-steroidal anti-inflammatory drugs.
   Corticosteroids.
   Polymyalgia rheumatica.
   Malignancy.
   Myelodysplastic syndrome.
b. Haematinic assays (serum ferritin, vitamin B_{12} and folate).
   Serum immunoglobulins and protein electrophoresis.
   Faecal occult bloods.
   Upper GIT tract endoscopy (if FOB positive).

This patient has a secondary anaemia, also termed anaemia of chronic disorders, which characteristically is normocytic, i.e. has an MCV within the normal range. If the illness resulting in the anaemia is prolonged, the red cells may become microcytic and the MCV thus drops below normal. The WBC is normal and the platelets are elevated at $567 \times 10^9/l$.

The differential diagnosis is wide and includes chronic infections (e.g. tuberculosis), inflammatory disorders (e.g. rheumatoid disease and other connective tissue disorders) and malignancy. Malignancy may be haematological (e.g. lymphoma, leukaemia or multiple myeloma) or non-haematological, such as carcinoma of bowel, breast, lung, etc. Another condition which may lead to this type of anaemia is chronic renal impairment. Bleeding must be considered especially in patients such as this, since she was on a combination of corticosteroids and a NSAID. In combination they increase the risk of gastric erosions. The elevated platelet count may reflect the reactive nature of the secondary anaemia or may suggest active bleeding. This type of anaemia may be seen in the elderly with long-term problems such as stasis ulcers, urinary infection, etc.

> The serum iron and TIBC are reduced but the serum ferritin is elevated (the latter being a reactive protein). The aetiology of the anaemia is unclear but may be mediated, in part, by IL-1. The overall result is ineffective iron utilization by developing red cells, also called reticuloendothelial iron block.

Efforts should be made to determine the cause of the anaemia and should include the investigations outlined above. If all the above investigations prove unhelpful, then it would be worth considering performing a bone marrow aspirate and trephine biopsy, which may distinguish the anaemia of chronic disorders from a myelodysplastic syndrome which is frequent in the elderly population.

Final diagnosis

Anaemia of chronic disorders. See Review articles.

Clinical case 3

a. Blood film examination.
   Full neurological examination to delineate the extent of the lesion(s) and determine the likely focus.
   Serum PSA.
   Autoimmune profile.
   CXR.
   CT of the brain.
   Consider Ham's test.
b. Occult malignancy with secondary deposits in the brain giving rise to the neurological symptoms and signs; demyelination; autoimmune disorder; cerebrovascular disease.

In a 59-year-old man with sudden onset of progressive neurological disease, degenerative disease and cancer are high on the list of diagnoses. The cancers most likely are lung, GI and prostate. Radiological investigations may help detect these, along with the serum PSA estimation. A primary neurological disease should be considered. In a patient of this age in western society cerebrovascular disease, i.e. stroke, should be considered.

However, straightforward cerebrovascular disease would not normally lead to the abnormal blood findings in this patient.

The blood film showed reduced neutrophils and platelets but no other diagnostic features. PSA was normal. Haematinics showed a normal serum B_{12} and red cell folate in addition to the elevated serum ferritin shown above. Ham's acid lysis test was performed to exclude paroxysmal nocturnal haemoglobinuria, a rare cause of pancytopenia. Biochemistry screen was unhelpful; thyroid function was normal. Autoimmune profile was negative. Blood was sent for immunological assessment of cell surface markers and revealed markedly reduced CD4 lymphocyte count ($<200/\mu l$).

Serology was unremarkable for *Mycoplasma*, Q fever, influenza A and B, adenovirus, measles, *Chlamydia* spp., RSV and CMV but did demonstrate definite evidence of infection by HIV.

Final diagnosis

CNS manifestations of HIV infection.

Clinical case 4

a. Malignancy such as lymphoma or acute leukaemia.
   Autoimmune disease, e.g. severe rheumatoid, SLE.
b. Autoimmune profile.
   CXR.
   Abdominal and pelvic ultrasound.
   Direct Coombs' test.
   Viral serology.
   Complement levels.
   Consider bone marrow aspirate and trephine biopsy.

This young woman has pancytopenia with reduction in haemoglobin, platelets and WBC. She also gives a history of weight loss of 15–20 kg over a short period of time. The other significant investigation findings include a grossly elevated ESR, CRP and serum ferritin. Whilst these are not diagnostic of any particular pathology, they do indicate severe underlying inflammation. The primary differential lies between a malignant process, e.g. Hodgkin's, NHL or acute leukaemia and connective tissue disease. Other causes of pancytopenia will need to be excluded.

Viral serology was essentially unhelpful with no evidence of parvovirus or hepatitis A, which might result in pancytopenia. The haematinics were normal thus excluding severe B_{12} or folate deficiency as a cause of pancytopenia; these would not give rise to the massively elevated CRP and ESR.

This patient was DCT-positive (IgA and IgG) but there was no evidence of underlying haemolysis (absent spherocytes, bilirubin normal, haptoglobins were present).

Autoimmune profile is useful to exclude or confirm connective tissue disease. In this case the results were as follows: thyroid microsomes, parietal cell, mitochondrial, skeletal muscle, smooth muscle and rheumatoid antibody screen was negative. Antinuclear antigen IgG showed a titre of 1 : 1024 and DNA binding was >300 i.u./ml. These were strongly suggestive of SLE. Complement levels were performed and these showed grossly reduced C3, C4 and a CH_{50} of <20% (normal range 80–120%). Radiological investigations were unhelpful. Bone marrow aspirate and trephine confirmed a hypocellular marrow with absence of erythroid cells, thus accounting for the profound anaemia.

The diagnosis in this case was SLE, a disorder of unknown aetiology characterized by production of autoantibodies with deposition of antibodies and immune complexes in tissues. B cell activity is increased, with antibodies produced against nuclear antigenic determinants. Clinical features are legion and include: rashes (sometimes butterfly rash on face), photosensitivity, myositis, alopecia, anaemia (± haemolysis), neutropenia, thrombocytopenia, lymphadenopathy, splenomegaly, cerebral disturbance including psychosis. Management is aimed at reducing inflammation and includes NSAIDs, corticosteroids, hydroxychloroquine and cytotoxics (e.g. cyclophosphamide). SLE may be controllable but is incurable.

Final diagnosis

SLE presenting with anaemia and leukopenia.

Clinical case 5

a. Peripheral blood film examination.
   Reticulocyte count.
   DAT.
   Peripheral blood cell markers (immunophenotype).
   Ultrasound scan of abdomen.
   CXR.
   Haematinic assays.

b. Leukaemia.
   Lymphoma.
   Haemolytic anaemia.

This man was profoundly anaemic on admission with indices that were highly abnormal: the MCV was grossly elevated at 130 fl and he had a raised WBC, most of which were reported by the automated counter as 'lymphocytes'. Anaemia with an MCV as high as this could be due to haematinic deficiency such as vitamin B_{12} or folate, but with this degree of anaemia his platelet and white cell counts would be expected to be lower. The reticulocytes were 33% (normal ≤2.5%) and since these cells are young red blood cells with a much higher MCV than normal mature RBCs, this would account for the grossly elevated MCV of 130 fl.

The DAT (direct Coombs') is used to detect the presence of antibodies on the red cell membrane. In this case the DAT was strongly positive and demonstrated the presence of IgG on the cell surface. This antibody was an autoantibody and the haemolytic anaemic process is therefore termed 'autoimmune haemolytic anaemia'. As part of the haemolysis the spleen removes the antibody coated red cells from the circulation prematurely and enlarges considerably in size.

> Examination of the peripheral blood film confirmed that the lymphocytes reported in the white cell differential were in fact abnormal lymphocytes resembling those found in lymphoma. Immunophenotyping confirmed these to be B cell in origin, making it highly likely that the patient had an underlying malignant B cell NHL. This accounted for the axillary node felt on initial examination. Production of paraproteins and autoantibodies is well described in a variety of lymphoid malignancies, including NHL.

The CXR was performed to determine whether there was any para-aortic lymphadenopathy or other pathology in the thorax. In this case the radiograph was normal. However, ultrasound examination of the patient's abdomen confirmed significant splenomegaly of 18 cm in length (normal ≤12 cm).

Final diagnosis

Autoimmune haemolytic anaemia secondary to underlying malignant B cell NHL.

Clinical case 6

a. Peripheral blood film examination.
   Blood films stained for malarial parasites.
   Full coagulation screen, including XDPs.
   Direct antiglobulin test.
   Autoantibody profile.
   Blood cultures.
b. Idiopathic thrombocytopenic purpura (ITP) with occult-bleeding.
   Thrombotic thrombocytopenic purpura (TTP).
   Disseminated intravascular coagulation (DIC).
   Systemic lupus erythematosus (SLE).
   Cerebral malaria.
   Sepsis, including meningitis.

The peripheral blood film demonstrated gross red cell fragmentation along with nucleated red blood cells and occasional myelocytes. The platelet numbers in the film were in agreement with the automated count. No malarial parasites were seen on either thick or thin films.

Coagulation tests were normal thus arguing against DIC. DAT and autoantibody profile were negative making SLE unlikely. Blood cultures demonstrated no growth.

The likeliest diagnosis was felt to be TTP, a disorder of unknown aetiology presenting with a classic pentad of fever, anaemia, thrombocytopenia, bizarre neurological features and renal failure. However, not all of these features may be present and, for example, in this case renal function was minimally affected. Occasionally there is a prodromal illness which may be suggestive of an infective aetiology but serological assays are inconsistent. The differential diagnosis must include: sepsis, DIC, bacterial endocarditis, SLE with CNS complications, PNH and metastatic cancer.

> TTP results in diffuse endothelial damage and disseminated platelet thrombi. Investigations should include: FBC (anaemia and severe thrombocytopenia, red cell fragments), WBC (elevated or normal) and clotting studies (normal). LDH will be elevated (haemolysis); microscopic haematuria, casts and proteinuria will be demonstrated; 50% of patients will have impaired renal function. The pathological lesions will show eosinophilic granular ('hyaline') material in the lumen of arterioles and capillaries made up, primarily, of platelets. Renal biopsy will demonstrate platelet and fibrin thrombi occluding glomerular capillary lumens.
>
> TTP may occur in pregnancy and is commoner in the second and third trimesters (HUS, in comparison, is commoner in the postpartum period). TTP/HUS may occur in conjunction with pre-eclampsia or in normal pregnancy. Distinction from PET may be difficult. Delivery may need to be carried out early if the patient is severely anaemic and/or thrombocytopenic. There is no risk of transmission to the baby and TTP may recur in future pregnancies.

This rare but devastating syndrome may overwhelm young adults and management consists of plasma exchange using fresh frozen plasma. The disorder carries a grave prognosis with a significant mortality rate even in the face of modern intensive management. Patients who respond to therapy may subsequently suffer a relapsing/remitting course requiring chronic intermittent plasma exchange for years. In spite of much research, no other effective therapies have been shown to be of consistent benefit.

Final diagnosis

TTP.

Clinical case 7

a. The FBC and reticulocyte count are entirely normal. Her ESR is mildly elevated at 23 mm/h, which would be in keeping with controlled RA. The clotting screen is essentially normal. More worrying is the IgG at 35 g/l, which is clearly outside the normal range. This may fit with RA or MS, depending on whether the IgG is polyclonal or clonal in nature (see below).

b. Electrophoretic strip is required in order to quantitate the IgG paraproteinaemia, if present. A rise in IgG of a polyclonal nature is seen in many infective or inflammatory processes. If, however, there is a monoclonal component in the IgG then this must be determined. In this patient the monoclonal IgG comprised ~50% of the total (i.e. 17–20 g/l) which does not fit with either RA or MS but rather suggests benign monoclonal gammopathy. Multiple myeloma may also give rise to elevated IgG to this extent and greater but this condition is unusual in a patient of this age since myeloma is typically a disorder of middle-aged/elderly people.

Full serum biochemistry profile is essential in order to check renal function and serum calcium level which may be abnormal in myeloma. The β_2-microglobulin should be checked. The skeletal survey should be reviewed for myelomatous lytic lesions present in a proportion of patients with myeloma.

A bone marrow aspirate and trephine biopsy should be obtained, seeking evidence for a rise in plasma cells. The marrow should be assessed by cell surface markers (flow cytometry), again looking for evidence of elevated plasma cell numbers and clonality. If a clonal population of plasma cells is present then most plasma cells will express κ or λ light chains on their cell surface since they will be derived from a single malignant cell. In health a mixture of light chains (i.e. κ and λ) is found in normal blood and marrow.

c. It would be prudent to 'watch and wait' and perform serial IgG levels with quantitation of paraproteinaemia, looking for a rise in the paraprotein suggestive of transformation of a benign paraprotein to a more aggressive disease, namely, multiple myeloma. This patient had an IgG of 20 g/l some 8 years previously which has been rising slowly over time. The IgG has, however, been stable for the past year or so and has never risen above the current level.

> There are three major groups of disorders characterized by production of paraprotein: MGUS, multiple myeloma and macroglobulinaemia. MGUS is found in 1% of the population >25 years of age, 3% >70 years and 10% >80 years. Diagnosis relies on immunoelectrophoresis for the detection of monoclonal immunoglobulin (M protein) in serum and urine. Fifty per cent of paraproteins are IgG, 20–25% are IgA, 15% are IgM and 10% are light chains only.
>
> Features suggestive of benign disease include: stable serum M protein over several years; M protein concentration <25 g/l; normal Igs are not suppressed; Bence Jones protein (urinary free light chains) is absent or only detectable in concentrated urine; plasma cells make up <10% nucleated cells in the marrow; β_2-microglobulin <2 mg/l.
>
> Some patients will progress from MGUS to florid myeloma and hence serial paraprotein levels need to be performed over several years in order to detect such progression.
>
> Serum β_2-microglobulin is the light chain of the MHC class I molecule, present on all nucleated cells. Where there is increased cell division (e.g. malignancy), there is increased turnover of β_2-microglobulin which is shed from cells. In myeloma, with renal impairment, the GFR falls and clearance of β_2-microglobulin is reduced. This leads to elevation of serum levels. β_2-microglobulin is a useful monitor of malignant cell mass, cell turnover, effect of tumours on renal function and response to therapy.

Final diagnosis

Benign paraproteinaemia/MGUS.

Clinical case 8

a. Causes of lymphadenopathy and weight loss in a young female: EBV.
   Lymphoma.
   Hodgkin's disease.
   HIV.
b. Viral serology, including EBV.
   Cell markers, including CD4 : CD8 ratio.
   Lymph node biopsy.
   Consider bone marrow examination.
   CT scan of the thorax/abdomen.

This question is aimed at investigation and management of lymphadenopathy in a young patient and examination candidates should be able to discuss this in MRCP and MRCPath examinations.

Consider other neck swellings: abscesses, infection in salivary glands, thyroid cysts and thyroglossal duct cysts. Posterior cervical glands: viral and bacterial infection, infectious mononucleosis, mycobacterial disease (tuberculous adenopathy), HIV infection, CMV, Hodgkin's, NHL, cat scratch fever, toxoplasmosis, histoplasmosis, occasionally drugs (pseudolymphoma with phenytoin; a small proportion of these eventually develop lymphoma), antithyroid drugs, isoniazid. Malignancies causing cervical lymphadenopathy include carcinomas, lymphoproliferative disease (Hodgkin's, non-Hodgkin's, ALL, CLL, etc.), head and neck tumours and breast cancer.

Final diagnosis

Hodgkin's disease.

Clinical case 9

a. Pancytopenia with splenomegaly.
   Need to consider:
   Carcinoma.
   Haemato-oncological disease, e.g. leukaemias, lymphomas (NHL, Hodgkin's disease, HCL and variant, CLL, splenic lymphoma with villous lymphocytes), myeloproliferative diseases (especially myelofibrosis).
b. You should ask for a blood film to be reviewed since we do not know what the 'atypical cells' were. Ask for the result of the bone marrow aspirate and trephine biopsy.
c. 2-CDA, 2-deoxycoformycin, interferon-α, splenectomy.
d. The prognosis is good; HCL is one of the low-grade lymphomas with long overall survival. In many cases, with the use of 2-CDA cure may be anticipated.

This patient was admitted with pneumonia, not unusual in itself. However, the FBC findings were highly abnormal with reduced Hb, WBC and platelets (i.e. pancytopenia). In a patient of this age carcinomas and lymphomas need to be excluded. Combined haematinic deficiency is possible but less likely. The FBC printout showed the presence of 'atypical cells', although we are not told what these were. A blood film should be examined, irrespective of these cells, in any patient with this type of blood picture. The biochemistry tests added little but the ultrasound was useful. This showed fatty infiltration (not unusual) and enlargement of the spleen, which is highly significant.

The medical team requested a bone marrow aspirate and trephine biopsy to exclude or confirm the presence of an under-lying malignant disease process. The aspirate was difficult (dry tap) but from the small amount of marrow that was obtained, some was sent for cell surface marker analysis. These showed that B cell markers predominate (CD19 and CD22) with predominance of κ, indicating that most B cells are expressing immunoglobulin of single specificity, suggesting the presence of a clone of cells. Normally a mixture of κ- and λ-expressing lymphocytes is present.

> Highly significant was the finding of 9% TRAP containing cells very suggestive of HCL. This was further supported by the marrow trephine whose appearance was consistent with a diagnosis of HCL. The TRAP test demonstrates the presence of an isoenzyme specific to hairy cells. Occasionally HCL is TRAP-negative (especially the HCL variant) and occasional cases of B cell prolymphocytic leukaemia or T cell lymphocytic leukaemia are TRAP-positive.
>
> HCL is a mature B cell neoplasm expressing B cell surface antigens but, unlike CLL, HCL expresses HC2. Whereas CLL cells are CD5 positive, HCL cells are always CD5-negative.
>
> Examination of the spleen shows diffuse infiltration of the splenic red pulp cords and sinuses by hairy cells.

Final diagnosis

Low-grade B cell lymphoproliferative disorder–HCL.

Clinical case 10

a. Marrow infiltration, e.g. leukaemia, lymphoma, myeloprolifer-ative disease, carcinoma.
b. The likeliest diagnosis is myeloproliferative disease and, in particular, myelofibrosis. This diagnosis is suggested by the high serum urate level (supporting the diagnosis of myelopro-liferative disease), progressive splenomegaly, weight loss and increased reticulin in the marrow.

Myelofibrosis is one distinct form of the myeloproliferative diseases. These are clonal neoplastic disorders of haematopoietic cells. The normal human marrow has little connective tissue; this is associated predominantly with trabecular surfaces. Increased reticulin is a consistent feature of myelofibrosis as well as fibrosis occurring as a secondary phenomenon (e.g. leukaemic infiltration, metastatic cancer in marrow, etc.).

Myelofibrosis mostly occurs in the middle-aged and elderly. There may be a prior history of polycythaemia rubra vera or essential thrombocythaemia. Patients present with symptoms and signs of progressive marrow failure (cytopenias, infections, bleeding) as well as constitutional symptoms (weight loss, sweats). The most prominent physical finding is splenomegaly, which may be massive. Lymph node enlargement is uncommon but is seen in some cases (extramedullary haematopoiesis).

> Haematological features include leukoerythroblastic anaemia (nucleated red cells and immature white cells in the peripheral blood) as well as teardrop cells. The patient often has a reduced haemoglobin and may have an associated reticulocytosis. The WBC may be elevated. The serum urate is elevated. Bone marrow aspirate is often unsuccessful (dry tap) but the trephine biopsy shows a gross increase in reticulin fibres.
>
> Median survival is around 5 years from diagnosis, although many patients survive >10 years. The commonest causes of death are infection and haemorrhage. Around 5–10% transform to AML.
>
> Treatment is essentially supportive with blood transfusion, allopurinol, and folic acid. Splenectomy is therapeutic for massive splenomegaly, excessive blood transfusion requirements and constitutional symptoms. There may be a role for drugs such as hydroxyurea depending on the WBC and degree of splenomegaly.

Final diagnosis

Idiopathic myelofibrosis.

Clinical case 11

a. Differential diagnosis would lie between myelomatosis and metastatic carcinoma of unknown primary.
b. Radiology: X-rays of her hip, pelvis and spine are indicated.
There were several small lytic lesions in her pelvis and a large lytic area in the left side of her pelvis in the area where she complained of pain. Generalized osteoporosis was noted. In addition to collapse of T12 there was also wedge collapse of L2 and L3 and lytic lesions noted in other vertebrae. A full skeletal survey was completed which showed other lytic lesions in her skull and upper femora.

Serum immunoglobulins demonstrated no monoclonal (M) bands. Total IgG was 2.6 g/l (normal 5.3–16.5 g/l), IgA was 0.2 g/l (normal 0.8–4.0 g/l) and IgM was <0.1 g/l (normal 0.5–2.0 g/l).

Urine was analysed for Bence Jones protein and was found to be negative. Serum β_2- microglobulin was estimated and found to be 3.8 mg/l. Bone marrow aspiration and biopsy were carried out; these showed extensive infiltration with atypical plasma cells indicative of multiple myeloma.

The diagnosis was, therefore, non-secretory myeloma. The commonest skeletal manifestation of multiple myeloma is osteoporosis, which can be severe and debilitating. Non-secretory myeloma accounts for 1% of the total cases of myeloma and frequently presents in this way. Investigation a year previously had been carried out to include immunoglobulin levels. These were done and were minimally reduced. Absence of a paraprotein was taken to exclude the diagnosis. Osteoporosis in isolation would not be an indication for bone marrow aspiration for suspected myeloma. A check on serum immunoglobulins would be advised to identify abnormal bands and screening for urinary immunoglobulin light chain excretion. Low levels of serum immunoglobulin should raise suspicion of either light chain or non-secretory myeloma which may otherwise be missed.

Final diagnosis

Non-secretory myeloma.

Clinical case 12

a. The likely diagnosis is an acute leukaemia. In this age group AML is more likely and the clinical events show a disproportionate bleeding diathesis, suggesting APML complicated by DIC as the most likely variant. Drug-related pancytopenia should be considered but neither of the agents quoted are typically associated with bone marrow problems. Diclofenac can cause a bleeding diathesis but this is mediated through interference with platelet function, not platelet numbers.

b. Detailed examination of her blood film showed an occasional circulating promyelocyte-like cell. Clotting tests were carried out. PT was 26 s (normal 12.0–14.0 s), partial thromboplastin time was 75 s (normal 26.0–33.5 s), thrombin clotting time was 20 s (normal 12–15 s). XDPs (fibrinogen degradation products) were >5000 μg/l (normal <250 μg/l). Fibrinogen was 1.2 g/l (normal 2.0–4.0 g/l). Urea, electrolytes and liver function tests were normal. Bone marrow examination was carried out; the marrow aspirate was difficult but showed marrow replacement with atypical promyelocytes with prominent granulation and numerous Auer rods. Cytogenetic analysis of the bone marrow showed the cells to contain the t(15;17) regarded as diagnostic of APML or AML M3 subtype.

c. Initial management involved confirmation of the diagnosis, supportive therapy with fresh frozen plasma and platelet concentrates together with full i.v. hydration. Once stabilized, chemotherapy was commenced using cytosine arabinoside, daunorubicin and thioguanine. She received additional ATRA in view of the diagnosis of APML.

> AML M3 is associated with a balanced chromosomal translocation between chromosomes 15 and 17, i.e. t(15;17). With rearrangement of DNA the chromosomal translocation produces two novel fusion genes involving PML and RARα: PML/RARα and RARα/PML. It is believed that the PML/RARα is responsible for the development of aberrant haematopoiesis. In fact, there are two isoforms of the PML/RARα fusion gene – long and short. Patients who possess the short isoform have a poorer clinical outcome than those in whom the long isoform is found but the exact mechanism involved is unclear at present. Abnormal expression of this gene correlates with responsiveness to ATRA, to which the leukaemic cells in AML M3 are exquisitely sensitive.
>
> The precise role of ATRA in the management of PML is being evaluated in clinical trials. On present data, the mortality during remission therapy in APML has not yet been reduced, as the major initial complication is haemorrhage from the DIC. Patients with APML and t(15;17) who achieve remission are now regarded as 'good-risk' patients with something like a 60% chance of staying in long-term remission. The presence of the fusion gene may be inferred from cytogenetic analysis (i.e. the presence of t(15;17)) or, more recently, by a RT-PCR method. In this, the PML/RARα mRNA is reverse-transcribed into cDNA, which is then used for PCR detection of the abnormal transcript. The PCR methodology has been used by several groups to monitor minimal residual disease in patients with treated AML M3.
>
> The mechanism of DIC in APML is not entirely known. Hypotheses include activation of the coagulation cascade directly by products from the malignant promyelocyte. An alternative explanation is the expulsion of procoagulant activity by reactive inflammatory cells and a third explanation is the possibility that the cell products may activate endothelial cells which then produce mediators of intravascular coagulation.
>
> See also Chapter 2, Figure 1.2.

Final diagnosis

AML M3 subtype (APML).

Clinical case 13

a. The likely cause of recurrent anaemia in this patient is recurrent iron deficiency. Previous data suggest a poor response to oral supplements but an unequivocal response to parenteral iron. Demonstration of a low ferritin confirmed the diagnosis of iron deficiency along with the pattern of response to i.v. iron.

b. Recurrent microcytic anaemia in this context must indicate recurrent iron deficiency. A ferritin confirmed this to be the case. Knowing that the haemoglobin had been normal 3 months previously indicates clearly that the patient was actively bleeding and that investigation must determine the site of blood loss and treat appropriately. Further relevant investigations must include a detailed repeat clinical history and examination. Factors such as NSAID ingestion, radical changes in menstruation or other forms of gynaecological blood loss were ruled out. On further questioning she admitted to variable degrees of abdominal distension and discomfort. Bowel habit had been modestly irregular and diet had been unchanged. Physical examination revealed only abdominal distension and some right iliac fossa tenderness.

FOBs were carried out and all three were positive. Gastroscopy and duodenal biopsy were normal.

Colonoscopy/barium enema appeared to be urgently indicated. Colonoscopy was carried out and suggested a lesion in the ascending colon; biopsy was suspicious of Crohn's disease. Follow-up barium enema indicated a large mass in the ascending colon.

Urea, electrolytes and liver function tests were all carried out and were unremarkable.

Ham's acid lysis test was carried out and was negative.

On the basis of the findings she proceeded to surgery. Resection of large bowel was carried out. The mass in the ascending colon was found to consist predominantly of Crohn's disease but there was a small area of adenocarcinomatous change present. She made an uneventful postoperative recovery and proceeded to have adjuvant chemotherapy. The diagnosis was made of recurrent refractory iron-deficiency anaemia secondary to occult GI blood loss from inflammatory bowel disease and neoplastic change.

Final diagnosis

Recurrent iron-deficiency anaemia secondary to underlying Crohn's disease and neoplastic change.

Clinical case 14

a. The problem is that of a young, previously fit man presenting with spontaneous bruising associated with thrombocytopenia and mild clotting abnormality. Clinical examination showed marked hepatosplenomegaly. Diagnostic possibilities include myeloproliferative disease or low-grade lymphoma/CLL. The association with abnormalities of clotting is unusual and points to an alternative diagnosis, in this case type 1 Gaucher's disease. This type of presentation is not atypical.
b. Bone marrow aspiration and biopsy. These showed prominent histiocytic infiltration indicating an underlying storage disorder. Further clotting tests indicated no deficiency of clotting factors but the presence of anticoagulant activity which could not be further defined. Such clotting abnormalities are described in Gaucher's disease. Measurement of leukocyte enzymes was arranged. This showed significant reduction in β-glucosidase activity, in keeping with the diagnosis of Gaucher's disease. Further molecular analysis was also carried out to demonstrate the specific type of Gaucher's mutation.

   Radiology was carried out; there were no focal bony abnormalities. There was marginal expansion in the distal femora suggestive of the 'Erlenmeyer flask' deformity characteristic of Gaucher's disease.
c. The patient was considered appropriate to receive Ceredase® therapy. This is enzyme replacement therapy specific for the condition and will produce regression of organomegaly and correction of bony abnormalities.

Type 1 Gaucher's disease is typically associated with a high incidence in Ashkenazi Jewish populations. However, there is an incidence of around 1:40 000 of the gene in the general population. It is not associated with any form of mental handicap or CNS manifestation and may be diagnosed at any time during life depending on severity. Some cases may not be identified until adult life. Indications for therapy would include organomegaly, abnormalities of clotting and extensive bony disease. Fortunately, the condition is still rare since therapy, although highly specific and effective, is expensive, with annual treatment costs estimated at around £75–£100 000 per annum.

> Gaucher's disease is an inherited disorder producing a deficiency in the enzyme glucocerebrosidase. In type 1 disease glycolipid accumulates in cells of the spleen, liver and bone marrow; in types 2 and 3 disease lipid accumulation is in brain cells. Type 2 disease produces severe progressive neurological deterioration from birth and is usually fatal within 1 year.

Presentation and severity of type 1 disease vary considerably between individual patients. The main clinical signs and symptoms include: (a) splenomegaly; (b) hepatomegaly; (c) anaemia, thrombocytopenia and bleeding abnormalities; (d) skeletal problems – failure of bone remodelling, osteopenia, osteonecrosis, osteosclerosis and bone crises characterized by acute episodes of severe bone pain.

Type 1 Gaucher's disease is a pan-ethnic disease, although the greatest predominance is seen in Ashkenazi Jews. Therapy previously was palliative and commonly included splenectomy. Severe cases have received allogeneic BMT.

Alglucerase is a modified form of human placental glucocerebrosidase that has been purified. In recent years it has been available for therapeutic usage; tissue infiltration and organomegaly due to Gaucher's disease have been reversed by regular infusions of alglucerase. A recombinant form of this enzyme may shortly be available for therapeutic use.

Therapeutic use of the enzyme has certainly improved symptoms and signs in many types of Gaucher's patients. Unfortunately, therapy is very expensive, with an annual cost in the order of £75 000.

Final diagnosis

Gaucher's disease.

Clinical case 15

a. Drug-induced pancytopenia.
   Rheumatoid disease/Felty's syndrome.
b. Bone marrow aspirate and trephine biopsy.
   Autoimmune profile.
   Screen for underlying malignancy (examination, CXR, FOBs, urinalysis, etc.).
c. Since her neutrophil count is $<1.0 \times 10^9/l$, it may be wise to consider a prophylactic antibacterial agent along with an antifungal since she has increased susceptibility to infection.
   Specific therapy is discussed below.

Acquired neutropenia may be due to drugs (predictable, e.g. cytotoxics, and idiosyncratic, e.g. NSAIDs, salicylates, antithyroid, etc.), infiltration of the marrow (carcinoma, leukaemia, lymphoma), secondary to infection (e.g. EBV, HIV) and nutritional deficiency (B_{12} or folate). There are several immune-mediated neutropenias as well as familial and cyclic forms.

Rather than neutropenia, however, this patient demonstrates pancytopenia with all three cell lines involved.

Rheumatoid disease and other connective tissue disorders could produce this blood picture but this woman's RA was mild and we know that the disease was not active (clinically, on examination and ESR). Felty's syndrome describes patients with RA, neutropenia and splenomegaly; splenomegaly was absent in this patient.

Various investigations were performed to determine whether her problems might be secondary to autoantibodies but none were detected.

In fact, this patient's problems were complex and investigation showed that she was suffering from LGL leukaemia, a disease also known as Tγ lymphocytosis or T-CLL.

> The diagnosis was made using a combination of peripheral blood cell markers and clonality studies using DNA probes for TCR genes. This patient's peripheral blood cell markers showed a predominance of CD3- and CD8-positive lymphocytes (T cells) with relative lack of B cells (CD19$^+$ cells). LGLs are one subset of normal circulating lymphocytes.
>
> The aetiology of the disease is unknown but EBV and retroviruses have been suggested as a cause in some cases. Clinical features are variable: patients tend to be elderly and suffer recurrent infection; rheumatoid is not uncommon. Patients often have splenomegaly, hepatomegaly, lymphadenopathy, skin and marrow infiltration.
>
> Typically the immunophenotype using cell markers is: CD3$^+$, CD4$^-$, CD8$^+$, CD16$^+$, CD56$^-$, TCRαβ$^+$ (occasionally TCRγδ$^+$).
>
> The main cause of morbidity and mortality is the neutropenia and infection is often the terminal event. Various treatments have been tried but there is no consensus regarding the best option. Treatments have included corticosteroids, splenectomy, methotrexate and recombinant human growth factors.

Final diagnosis

RA and LGL leukaemia.

Clinical case 16

a. Chronic liver disease (cirrhosis) secondary to alcohol, viral hepatitis or autoimmune disease.
Porphyria cutanea tarda.
Hereditary 'idiopathic' haemochromatosis.
b. Abdominal ultrasound.
Autoimmune profile.
Serology for evidence of hepatitis B and C.
Urinary porphyrin excretion and faecal isocoproporphyrin estimation.
Serum iron and TIBC.
Liver biopsy for histology and assessment of iron content.

Macrocytosis is a common feature of liver disease, especially that associated with alcohol ingestion. Serum vitamin B_{12} may be raised in liver disease, sometimes as a result of increased levels of transcobalamin II.

The diagnosis in this case was hereditary haemochromatosis. The serum iron was 32 μmol/l (normal range 14–33 μmol/l) and the TIBC was 33 μmol/l (normal range 45–75 μmol/l), thus reflecting a transferrin saturation of close to 100%. The inheritance is typically autosomal recessive and the disease usually presents in the fifth decade or later with a male predominance. Apart from diabetes mellitus, iron deposition may result in a number of endocrinopathies (e.g. hypothyroidism, hypothalamic pituitary insufficiency and hypogonadism). Deposition in heart muscle may result in a variety of cardiac abnormalities, such as arrhythmias and congestive failure. The typical skin hyperpigmentation results mainly from melanin deposition and results in the syndrome of 'bronzed diabetes'. In the absence of treatment, the liver disease progresses to cirrhosis and hepatocellular carcinoma develops in up to 30% of cases (the brother of this patient died of hepatoma).

Diagnosis of hereditary haemochromatosis requires a high index of clinical suspicion and screening tests for iron overload. If the serum iron concentration exceeds 35 μmol/l and the transferrin saturation is greater than 60%, then haemochromatosis is likely in the absence of other obvious causes of iron loading. The serum ferritin is typically greater than 500 μg/l and often exceeds 1000 μg/l.

> Venesection remains the mainstay of therapy and may have to be repeated weekly or twice weekly for 1–2 years in order to remove excess iron load. Chelating agents such as desferrioxamine may also help to reduce the iron overload but are very expensive and seldom used. Additional therapeutic measures include the management of diabetes and cardiac arrhythmias and insufficiency. Hepatocellular failure and cirrhosis require supportive care and it is vital to avoid alcohol and other hepatotoxins.

Final diagnosis

Hereditary haemochromatosis.

Clinical case 17

a. MDS.
   Other causes of pancytopenia should be considered (e.g. drugs, infections, infiltrations).
b. Treatment is essentially supportive with blood and platelet transfusions as required to control symptoms. Antibiotic prophylaxis may be useful when significant neutropenia is a feature (e.g. $<0.5 \times 10^9/l$).
c. The prognosis varies with the subtype of MDS. Refractory anaemia and refractory anaemia with ring sideroblasts have the best prognosis.

The MDSs represent a group of clonal haematopoietic cell disorders which range from mild abnormalities in haematopoietic cell production to overt pre-leukaemic changes. Typically, MDS occurs in middle-aged or elderly patients, although childhood forms do exist. Clinical manifestations are those of impaired marrow function, although only one effect, e.g. anaemia or neutropenia, may predominate.

Classification

Refractory anaemia	RA
Refractory anaemia with ring sideroblasts	RARS
Refractory anaemia with excess blasts	RAEB
Refractory anaemia with excess blasts in transformation	RAEB-t
Chronic myelomonocytic leukaemia	CMML

Management is supportive; intensive chemotherapy is not appropriate in most cases. A small proportion of younger patients with RAEB-t may benefit from AML-type therapy approaches involving intensive chemotherapy.

Myelodysplasia is discussed in detail in the Review articles. (Chapter 7).

Final diagnosis

Myelodysplastic syndrome.

Clinical case 18

a. Serum ferritin.
   Possibly iron and TIBC.
   Upper GI tract endoscopy and perhaps colonoscopy.
   Gynaecological review.
   Consider FOBs.
b. A reduced haemoglobin and MCV in a young woman with heavy periods suggests iron-deficiency anaemia. The bruising is not significant in this case and the lymph nodes were small and not suggestive of any serious underlying pathology.
c. (i) Elimination of the cause (menorrhagia needs to be controlled; in this case the oral contraceptive pill was started which reduced the severity of bleeding in this patient).
   (ii) Simple iron supplements, e.g. ferrous sulphate 200 mg t.d.s.

This patient appeared to have a complicated history but after reviewing the FBC and the history of menorrhagia it was clear that this woman had iron-deficiency anaemia. The nodes and other aspects of the history proved not relevant.

Serum ferritin was checked and found to be 4 μg/l (normal range 14–200 μg/l). For some reason, iron and TIBC were also checked (unnecessary since the ferritin gave the diagnosis) and the iron was found to be low at 3 μmol/l (normal 11–28 μmol/l) and TIBC elevated at 89 μmol/l (normal 45–75 μmol/l): again, very much in keeping with simple iron deficiency. FOBs were checked and these were negative. An abdominal ultrasound was performed to exclude fibroids and this was entirely normal apart from a 'floppy collecting system' in the right kidney, felt to be due to 'post-pregnancy changes'. A CXR was normal.

She was started on iron and a low-dose contraceptive pill and her haematological indices returned to normal within a month. She was advised to take iron for 4 months in order to replenish her iron stores.

Final diagnosis

Iron-deficiency anaemia secondary to menorrhagia.

Clinical case 19

a. This patient presented with a severe pancytopenia. With this severity the diagnosis is likely to be either severe marrow aplasia or an acute leukaemia with an aleukaemic presentation. A high-grade lymphoma or other carcinomata might rarely present in this way; however, aplasia and leukaemia are by far the most likely.

b. A repeat blood count with film examination including reticulocyte count should be carried out. This confirmed severe pancytopenia and a virtual absence of reticulocytes, indicating profound marrow failure. Careful scrutiny of the film showed no circulating blast cells and bone marrow aspirate and biopsy were performed urgently. Aspirate material contained only a few particles which were grossly hypocellular. Trephine biopsy showed severe aplastic change.

c. Immediate management of the problem is to treat severe infection in a patient with bone marrow failure. CXR, blood cultures and an MSU should all be carried out in an attempt to identify the likely organism. Most commonly no specific pathogen is identified and the patient requires management with empirical i.v. antibiotics. Combined therapy with an aminoglycoside (e.g. gentamicin) and a ureidopenicillin (e.g. azlocillin) would be the most commonly used first-line antibiotics. Single-agent ceftazidime could equally well be used. The patient also requires full supportive therapy with i.v. hydration, mouth care and supportive transfusion.

In planning transfusion therapy the likely underlying diagnosis of severe aplasia or a leukaemia should be apparent early on. At 37, such a patient would be a candidate for bone marrow allografting (or autografting in a leukaemic situation). In this setting, transfused blood should be CMV-negative until the patient's CMV status is known. It should be leucodepleted to keep sensitization to foreign antigens at a minimum. In an emergency, however, this course of action may be impracticable. The immediate management is designed to contain the infective problem and allow the patient to survive so that the diagnosis can be clarified and appropriate therapy applied.

The diagnosis in this patient was severe aplastic anaemia secondary to hepatitis A infection. Aplastic anaemia is rare and is usually truly idiopathic. Other causes include drug idiosyncrasy; it is a rare occurrence following hepatitis A infection.

Post-hepatitic aplastic anaemia is a very severe form of aplastic anaemia with a high mortality. The patient falls into the category of severe aplastic anaemia on the basis of platelets <20 × 10^9/l and circulating neutrophils <0.5 × 10^9/l. Allogeneic BMT would be the treatment of choice in this individual if a donor were available. In the absence of a donor very encouraging results are obtained with high-dose steroids allied to the use of antithymocyte globulin. This patient did have an allogeneic sibling donor and, after stabilizing his marrow aplasia, BMT was carried out. Initial progress was encouraging but at 3 weeks graft-versus-host complications occurred in the skin, GI tract and liver. These could not be controlled and the patient died from GVHD.

Final diagnosis

Post-hepatitic aplastic anaemia.

Clinical case 20

a. Monospot test was negative.

Viral serology

EBV, toxoplasma and CMV antibody tests were negative.
Complement fixation tests for antibodies to other agents, including adenovirus, measles, *Mycoplasma* and influenza were also negative.

HIV serology

This was performed and she was found to be HIV-antibody-positive. p24 antigen was positive.

Lymph node biopsy

This showed reactive follicular hyperplasia with no evidence of NHL.

Immunoglobulin quantitation

A polyclonal increase in IgG was noted. Total IgG was 32.8 g/l (normal range 5.3–16.5 g/l). No monoclonal bands were present.

Lymphocyte subsets

This showed a significant diminution of absolute CD4 count and an increase in CD8 count. There was no clonal lymphocytosis.

Bone marrow aspirate and trephine biopsy

These were normal with no diagnostic features.
Bone marrow aspirate and biopsy were undertaken, aspirate and biopsy were normal with no diagnostic features.

b. Differential diagnoses: lymphoma (Hodgkin's or NHL); persistent viral infection or persistent generalized lymphadenopathy of HIV infection; acute presentation of a collagen disorder.

> This patient presented with non-specific symptoms and lymphadenopathy. She was initially thought to have lymphoma as no apparent risk factors for HIV infection were present on initial assessment. The absence of antibodies to common causes of glandular-fever-like illness and the lymph node appearances led to the suspicion of HIV infection, which was confirmed on subsequent testing.
>
> A patient presenting with persistent cytopenia, raised ESR, and fluctuating generalized lymphadenopathy should certainly be suspected of having HIV infection. Haematological manifestations of HIV infection include leukopenia and lymphopenia. Mild degrees of thrombocytopenia may be present although quite severe degrees of thrombocytopenia also occur in HIV infection. Polyclonal increase in immunoglobulins is common.
>
> Review of the history showed no obvious risk factors in the lifestyle of the young woman but her fiancé had been infected through a homosexual assault some years previously.

Final diagnosis

HIV infection.

Clinical case 21

a. The clinical features are most suggestive of an acute form of RA or other collagen disorder. The features could also be a presentation of an acute leukaemia or myelodysplasia.
b. A repeat blood count and film were requested. This confirmed the findings and no blast cells were seen on the blood film. Bone marrow aspiration and biopsy would be appropriate. These were carried out and showed normal maturation and development of all cell lines. Marrow cellularity was normal on the biopsy with no lymphomatous or other infiltrates. An autoimmune profile was carried out. Rheumatoid ELISA was positive at 200 i.u./l. Antinuclear factor was positive, IgG antibodies negative, IgM titre 1 : 160.

CRP was elevated at 82.3 mg/l (normal <6.0 mg/l). Urea and electrolytes were normal. Liver function tests were carried out and were normal apart from a marginal serum albumin of 30 g/l. Temporal artery biopsy was carried out and was normal. C3 and C4 complement levels were normal.

The patient was considered to have an acute form of rheumatoid/SLE. She was treated with steroids and the peripheral blood counts improved rapidly and symptoms were eased. She pursued a relapsing and remitting course over the next 2–3 years.

Severe cytopenia is a rare presentation of autoimmune disorders. In RA severe neutropenia may occur in Felty's syndrome; this is normally in the presence of a clearly palpable spleen. Autoimmune haemolysis and thrombocytopenia can occur in SLE as well as autoimmune granulocytopenia. Looking for granulocyte antibodies is not a wholly satisfactory diagnostic test, although evidence of reacting antibodies may be found. The principal function in investigation and management is to distinguish between a collagen disorder requiring steroid or other immunosuppressive therapy and an acute presentation of a haematological malignancy.

Final diagnosis

Active RA.

Clinical case 22

a. More details are required relating to the GI symptoms, e.g. When is the patient nauseous? How long has this been going on? Is there associated abdominal pain? Are there alterations in bowel habit? What is the degree of weight loss? Is there vomiting and haematemesis? Elicit details of the past medical history and drug ingestion.
b. The patient was anaemic with GI symptoms. The ferritin was normal but may be spuriously so, since the ESR was elevated. She also had liver function disturbance and profound hypoalbuminaemia. Initial investigations should be gastroenterological and should include upper GI tract endoscopy, abdominal ultrasound (looking for hepatosplenomegaly, lymph nodes, metastases). CXR is mandatory in a patient of this age, especially with these symptoms.
c. Cholestasis.
   Metastatic carcinoma.
   Hepatocellular carcinoma.

In light of the deranged LFTs and clinical picture of worsening jaundice this woman underwent ERCP which showed a normal bile duct but the presence of a large gastric ulcer on the lesser curve with evidence of recent bleeding. Furthermore, the ulcer appeared neoplastic and six biopsies were taken. The histology confirmed adenocarcinoma.

Gastric carcinoma may be insidious with relatively few symptoms. By the time patients present, the disease may have spread beyond the primary site to a distant site, e.g. liver, lungs, marrow.

Predisposing factors for gastric cancer include patients of blood group A, previous adenomatous polyps, PA, dermatomyositis and Barrett's oesophagus.

Final diagnosis

Adenocarcinoma (gastric) with liver metastases.

Clinical case 23

a. Alternative explanations for this persistent microcytic anaemia must include chronic disorder anaemia which can produce a significant microcytosis on occasions and also an underlying haemoglobin disorder such as β-thalassaemia trait. However, the Hb in this case is a little too low for thalassaemia trait to be a likely cause; more usually, the Hb is between 9.5–12.0 g/dl in a male.
b. Further investigations should include the following:
  (i)   Serum ferritin: this was done and was found to be 193 μg/l.
  (ii) Hb electrophoresis may be helpful; this was carried out and no evidence of thalassaemia trait was identified.
  (iii) Bone marrow examination: this would definitively assess iron stores. Marrow aspirate showed marked reactive change, satisfactory maturation of all normal elements and increased reticuloendothelial iron.
  (iv) Autoimmune profile: this was carried out to determine if there was any serological evidence of an underlying collagen disorder; all tests were negative.
  (v)   CXR: this was done by the GP initially and was normal. A repeat CXR on referral was also normal.
  (vi) Ultrasound: because of the finding of a chronic disorder anaemia, abdominal and pelvic ultrasound were carried out looking for occult malignancies. Evidence of a left renal mass was noted on ultrasound. Follow-up IVU and angiography confirmed the presence of a likely renal tumour. This was resected and a well-differentiated adeno-carcinoma was identified. The patient made an uneventful postoperative recovery and FBC normalized.

The diagnosis in this case was of a chronic disorder anaemia secondary to an underlying renal carcinoma. Initial investigation indicated a low serum iron not accompanied by a significant elevation of the TIBC. It is only the combination of reduced serum iron and raised TIBC that is diagnostic of iron-deficiency anaemia. Non-responsiveness to therapeutic doses of iron also clearly focused on alternative causes for the anaemia.

> The patient was of British ancestry and the finding of a normal FBC on BUPA screening over a year previously made a haemoglobin disorder extremely unlikely. In the absence of evidence of chronic infection or a collagen disorder an occult neoplasm seemed likely. Imaging techniques were employed to identify any possible primary site and the initial investigation with abdominal ultrasound revealed the cause. Chronic disorder anaemia usually has a normal or minimally reduced MCV, but in up to 30% of cases it may be markedly reduced.
>
> The mechanism of chronic disorder anaemia is not fully understood. There does appear to be both a reduction in the output of erythropoietin to compensate for the presence of the anaemia as well as a reduction in responsiveness of the marrow cells to erythropoietin itself. This appears to be mediated by a variety of cytokines, of which IL-1 appears to play a key role. This may be a mediator to release inhibitory factors such as interferon-γ from T lymphocytes, an interferon-β from marrow stromal cells to produce the chronic anaemia.

Secondary anaemia (chronic disorder anaemia) is discussed in the Review articles (chapter 7).

Final diagnosis

Anaemia of chronic disorders.

Clinical case 24

a. The differential diagnosis in a patient with known myelofibrosis would include myelofibrotic change in the lymph node or leukaemic infiltration. Such features do occur in the course of myeloproliferative disease. Features could represent an alternative malignancy such as metastatic carcinoma. Although he had been a non-smoker he had worked in a cable manufacturing plant and may well have been exposed to carcinogens. Infective causes should also be suspected: in a man of 75 with a haematological malignancy who has recently had steroids, tuberculous infection should be suspected.

b. Several investigations were performed: a CXR demonstrated enlargement of the mediastinum which had not previously been seen on earlier views. Blood cultures were negative. A biopsy of the node was arranged. Biopsy revealed necrotic, purulent material. No satisfactory histology was obtained. Microbiology smears were prepared which showed extensive neutrophil infiltration and a few acid-fast organisms. Review of the diagnostic material relating to the diagnosis of myelofibrosis was instituted. Peripheral blood and marrow changes were entirely consistent with myelofibrosis. Cytogenetics had been performed on the initial marrow sample with a karyotypic abnormality, 9p$^+$, described. The small number of blast cells were marked with CD13 indicative of early myeloid origin. Non-caseating granulomata were present on the original biopsy and had been judged as consistent with underlying myelofibrosis with no reason to suspect tuberculous infection.

The patient went on to receive antituberculous therapy without any major symptomatic benefit. His myelofibrotic condition remained active and shortly afterwards he developed portal vein thrombosis. Despite on-going supportive therapy, the patient died some 6 months later.

The initial presentation in this case was reasonably typical of cellular phase myelofibrosis. The findings of a leukocytosis, blood film abnormalities, accompanied by hepatosplenomegaly with weight loss and night sweats were fully supportive. This type of myelofibrotic presentation can be initially confused with CML. The total white count is usually not so high and the differential white cell appearances are different. In CML the complete range of maturation is seen and basophilia is prominent. Cytogenetics are usually advisable to distinguish the two conditions. The identification of a separate karyotypic abnormality, 9p$^+$, confirmed an underlying marrow problem and excluded CML.

> Cytotoxic therapy can be tried in myelofibrosis to reduce cellular proliferation and control symptoms. Splenectomy in myelofibrosis is helpful as a symptomatic measure; survival is not prolonged after the procedure but it can be very effective at reducing constitutional symptoms, discomfort from a massively enlarged spleen and transfusion dependency. Non-specific measures such as steroid therapy should be used very sparingly. The association between tuberculous infection and haematological malignancy is not entirely clear: there does appear to be an increased incidence of active tuberculous infection in patients with haematological disorders, perhaps due to underlying compromised immunity. It is difficult to diagnose. In addition to *Mycobacterium tuberculosis* other forms of mycobacterial infection may occur in haematological malignancy, notably forms such as *M. kansasii* in HCL. Tuberculous infection is also increased in HIV positive patients.

Final diagnosis

Myelofibrosis and tuberculosis.

Clinical case 25

a. EBV infection.
Toxoplasma infection.
Other viral infection, e.g. HIV.
Acute leukaemia.

b. Viral titres were carried out and these confirmed evidence of past EBV infection. The symptoms and signs were non-specific. No clear risk factors for HIV were identified but in the presence of leukopenia and mild thrombocytopenia it was felt appropriate to carry out a test after obtaining his consent. The HIV test proved negative. Because of persisting cytopenia associated with non-specific symptoms, including some bone discomfort, an autoimmune profile was undertaken. Rheumatoid factor was negative, ANA was negative and all other autoantibody testing proved similarly negative.

In view of the pancytopenia and persistent symptoms imaging of the chest and abdomen was undertaken. CXR was normal; abdominal ultrasound showed no lymphadenopathy but a minimal degree of splenomegaly. In view of his persisting symptoms, bone marrow aspirate was recommended and performed. This showed extensive infiltration with leukaemic cells. Cytochemistry indicated these cells to be negative with Sudan black and esterase stains. Cell surface markers showed the characteristic phenotype of HLA class II$^+$, TdT$^+$, CD10$^+$ indicative of common ALL.

He was advised appropriately and chemotherapy was given in accordance with the current Medical Research Council UK ALL protocol. He achieved a complete remission; there were no HLA-compatible family siblings and he was thus not eligible for allogeneic transplantation. After achieving remission, CNS prophylaxis was given and then 18 months of maintenance chemotherapy. He remains presently in first complete remission.

Presentation of acute leukaemia can be very dramatic or it may have a longer prodrome, as in this case. Symptoms can be entirely non-specific; clinical suspicion was alerted by the finding of persisting, unexplained neutropenia and a gradual evolution of mild anaemia and thrombocytopenia. The occurrence of a recent viral infection was almost certainly a coincidence in this case but created difficulty as many of his symptoms could equally well have been attributed to the post viral fatigue syndrome. Usually there are no haematological abnormalities in the post viral fatigue syndrome and persistence of haematological abnormalities must always be viewed with suspicion and concern.

In younger adults the commonest form of acute leukaemia remains AML, but up to 25% of cases may be ALL. Prognosis for ALL in younger adults is much less satisfactory than that for children with favourable risk factors. Current estimations for curability with existing treatment protocols suggest a 30–45% 5-year relapse-free survival. Adverse prognostic features include male sex, high presenting total WBC, hypodiploid karyotypic abnormalities and the presence of the Philadelphia chromosome.

Final diagnosis

Adult common acute lymphoblastic leukaemia (cALL).

5 Data interpretation questions

Data interpretation 1

A 26-year-old female shop assistant presented with recent onset of malaise and sweats. She was generally fit and well and her past medical history was unremarkable.

On examination there were a few shotty glands in the cervical area and her spleen was just palpable and moderately tender. Hepatomegaly was not detected. Her GP performed an FBC and initial biochemistry investigations, the results of which were as follows:

Hb 11.5 g/dl
WBC 14.3 × 10^9/l
neutrophils 1.1 × 10^9/l
lymphocytes 12.5 × 10^9/l
platelets 75 × 10^9/l

serum urea 4.5 mmol/l
serum creatinine 80 μmol/l
serum potassium 4.1 mmol/l
serum alanine aminotransferase 60 i.u./l

a. What further investigations would you perform?
b. Briefly discuss the differential diagnoses.

Data interpretation 2

A 56-year-old man presented to his GP with a 7-day history of increasing lassitude, intermittent backache and rigors. His past medical history included a hernia repair 10 years previously; there was nothing else of note. He was on no regular medication and had last consulted his GP 5 years before, following a respiratory infection. Pallor was noted on clinical assessment; BP was 125/85 mmHg and pulse 100 beats/min and regular. Axillary temperature was 37.6°C. He was referred for a blood count to the local hospital; after venepuncture he had a syncopal episode and was admitted as an emergency for observation.

No specific findings were identified on admission other than pallor, mild icterus and tachycardia. Abdominal examination was normal; rectal examination was unremarkable with normal stool colour.

Investigations on admission showed:

Hb 8.9g/dl
MCV 96 fl
WBC 9.2 × 10^9/l
platelets 387 × 10^9/l

Blood film comment: normochromic red cells, occasional frag-mented red cells noted and some polychromasia; white blood cells and platelets appear normal.

a. Suggest a likely cause for the findings described.
b. List four appropriate investigations likely to assist immediate diagnosis and further management.

Data interpretation 3

A 10-year-old girl was seen by the school doctor after she noticed large bruises on her shins appearing after a netball game. A family history was unremarkable. Apart from moderate bleeding following a dental extraction 1 year previously, the patient was otherwise fit and well.

An FBC and clotting screen revealed:

Hb 12.2 g/dl
WBC 6.7 × 10^9/l
platelets 205 × 10^9/l

PT 13 s (normal range 12.0–14.0 s)
APTT 48 s (normal range 26.0–33.5 s)
fibrinogen 3.2 g/l (normal range 2.0–4.0 g/l)

a. What other investigations are indicated in this patient?
b. What is the likely cause for her bruising?

Data interpretation 4

A 16-year-old female with lassitude was seen by her GP who performed an FBC which showed:

Hb 8.3 g/dl
MCV 65 fl

MCH 20 pg
MCHC 26 g/dl

a. Give two possible causes for these findings.
b. What further investigations would you request?

Data interpretation 5

A 69-year-old man presented to his family doctor with recurrent respiratory tract infections and troublesome epistaxes. An FBC was performed and this showed:

Hb 10.5 g/dl
MCV 90 fl
WBC 3.4 × 10^9/l
neutrophils 1.2 × 10^9/l
platelets 19 × 10^9/l

PT 14 s (normal range 12.0–14.0 s)
APTT 36 s (normal range 26.0–33.5 s)

a. What three further urgent investigations would you organize?
b. What two diagnoses would fit these data?

Data interpretation 6

James, a 22-year-old trainee estate agent, was admitted for minor elective surgery for a testicular hydrocele. Immediately postoperatively he complained of severe pain and discomfort in the wound. Inspection revealed a large haematoma and massive scrotal swelling.

He had previously been well with no known medical problems. He was on no regular medication. The bleeding was not thought to be surgical. A blood count and clotting screen were urgently requested, the results of which showed:

Hb 12.5 g/dl
MCV 87 fl
WBC 5.3 × 10^9/l
platelets 325 × 10^9/l

PT 13 s (normal range 12.0–14.0 s)
APTT 94 s (normal range 26.0–33.5 s)
fibrinogen 3.2 g/l (normal range 2.0–4.0 g/l)

a. Suggest a likely diagnosis for the these findings and results.
b. Specify three further investigations to make the diagnosis.
c. Suggest appropriate immediate management.

Data interpretation 7

A 13-year-old girl was referred because of heavy periods which
had been a feature since the menarche two years previously. She
had suffered from occasional troublesome nosebleeds in infancy,
but had otherwise been well. There was no family history of a
bleeding tendency.
    Investigations were performed as follows:

Hb 10.0 g/dl
PCV 0.32
MCV 72 fl
MCH 25 pg
MCHC 29 g/dl
WBC 9.6 × 10⁹/l
platelets 410 × 10⁹/l

blood film: hypochromic microcytic cells

serum ferritin 6 µg/l (normal range 14–200 µg/l)

PT 20 s (normal range 12.0–14.0)
APTT 48 s (normal range 26.0–33.5 s)
thrombin time 29 s (normal range 12.0–18.0 s)
reptilase time 35 s (normal range 12.0–18.0 s)
fibrinogen (Clauss) 0.4 g/l (normal range 2.0–4.0 g/l)
fibrinogen/fibrin degradation products <10 µg/ml (normal <10
µg/ml)
cross-linked fibrin D-dimers <250 mg/l (normal <250 mg/l)

a. What is the cause of her presenting symptoms?
b. What has been the result of this?
c. What further investigations are indicated?
d. How would you manage this patient?

Data interpretation 8

A 34-year-old journalist was admitted unconscious to the Accident & Emergency department. Initial examination revealed no evidence of head injury and no focal neurological signs were found. An FBC showed:

Hb 7.4 g/dl
MCV 123 fl
WBC 10.4 × 10^9/l
platelets 115 × 10^9/l

Blood film report: oval macrocytes and hypersegmented neutrophils noted; platelets are moderately reduced on the film.

a. What is the likely diagnosis?
b. What investigations would you perform?
c. Discuss the management.

Data interpretation 9

A 43-year-old woman was admitted to hospital with suspected DVT. She had two normal pregnancies several years before and was otherwise in good health and was receiving no regular medication. Over the past month she had suffered mild backache and had lost 2 kg in weight. She gave no history of night sweats or alteration in bowel habit but did admit to mild pruritus.
   An FBC showed:

Hb 8.5 g/dl
WBC 10.2 × 10^9/l
neutrophils 7.9 × 10^9/l
lymphocytes 2.1 × 10^9/l
platelets 1105 × 10^9/l

blood film report: rouleaux, thrombocytosis and occasional myelocyte seen

a. What are the differential diagnoses?
b. What further investigations are indicated?

Data interpretation 10

A 20-year-old Jamaican woman was admitted to hospital with pains in her arms and legs with associated fever. This apparently began after an exercise class. On admission she was obviously uncomfortable. Her axillary temperature was 38°C. There were few physical findings apart from a few coarse inspiratory crepitations in the left mid-zone. During the consultation she volunteered that she may have sickle cell trait but was unsure. Both parents, she thought, had sickle trait.

Investigations showed:

Hb 10.4 g/dl
MCV 71 fl
RCC $4.67 \times 10^{12}/l$
WBC $7.2 \times 10^9/l$
neutrophils $4.9 \times 10^9/l$
platelets $195 \times 10^9/l$

Film comment: target cells, coarse basophilic stippling, slight increase in polychromasia, occasional sickled cells noted.

Haemoglobin electrophoresis:
HbA	19.8%
HbA$_2$	5.5%
HbS	73.2 %
HbF	1.5%

a. What was the principal event underlying the hospital admission?
b. Interpret the haemoglobin electrophoretic results.
c. How would you manage this patient in the short and long term?

Data interpretation 11

A 67-year-old retired farmer presented to his family doctor with recurrent rectal bleeding over the past 3 months. On occasions his haemoglobin dropped to less than 10 g/dl, requiring admission for blood transfusion. He had no past history of serious illnesses and he was taking no medication regularly, apart from cod liver oil capsules. On examination he was noted to be pale but with no evidence of jaundice, clubbing or lymphadenopathy. Abdominal examination was normal.

Initial clotting results showed:

PT 14.0 s (normal range 12.0–14.0 s)
APTT 45.4 s (normal range 26.0–33.5 s)
thrombin time 15.6 s (control 16.1 s)
fibrinogen 2.7 g/l (normal range 2.0–4.0 g/l)
bleeding time 8 min (normal 3–9 min)

Based on these tests, further clotting tests were arranged, in which the patient's plasma was mixed with a variety of other plasmas:

APTT 50:50 control: patient plasma 37 s
APTT 50:50 aged normal serum: patient plasma 43 s
APTT 50:50 adsorbed plasma: patient plasma 30 s

a. What do these results suggest?
b. What further investigations would you perform?
c. How would you manage this patient?

Data interpretation 12

A 66-year-old retired car mechanic presented to his GP with a 6-month history of fatigue. During the previous month he had noticed increasing breathlessness on exertion. He also described night sweats occurring 2 or 3 times per week during the previous 3 months.

Previously he had been well; he was on no regular medication. His past history consisted only of a herniorrhaphy 7 years before. He was a non-smoker with an alcohol intake of 21 units per week.

Clinical examination showed pallor. His pulse was 84 beats/min and regular. There was no lymphadenopathy; the spleen was enlarged and palpable 4 cm below the costal margin.

Investigations showed:

Hb 6.2 g/dl
WBC 10.0 × 10^9/l
platelets 115 × 10^9/l
ESR >150 mm/1st hour (Westergren)

blood film: rouleaux, ~30% of white cells are atypical lymphocytes

serum sodium 131 mmol/l
serum potassium 3.5 mmol/l
serum urea 8.2 mmol/l
serum creatinine 116 μmol/l
serum total protein 120 g/l

a. What further investigations would be useful?
b. What is this patient's likely diagnosis?
c. Outline your management of this patient.

Data interpretation 13

A 57-year-old woman was referred to a cardiologist by her GP since she had been suffering palpitations associated with difficulty breathing intermittently for several weeks. Her past medical history was unremarkable and examination of the patient showed no abnormal findings. She was an ex-smoker of 4 months.

A variety of blood tests were arranged, the results of which were as follows:

Hb 11.5 g/dl
MCV 96.6 fl
WBC 9.0×10^9/l
neutrophils 5.4×10^9/l
platelets 1578×10^9/l

coagulation screen – normal

urea and electrolytes – normal
serum calcium 2.59 mmol/l
serum albumin 53 g/l

a. List six possible causes for these findings.
b. Which do you think is the likeliest?
c. What further investigations would you organize?
d. How would you manage this patient?

Data interpretation 14

A 36-year-old man was admitted to hospital acutely unwell with shortness of breath and haemoptysis. Investigations confirmed DVT with pulmonary embolism. On direct questioning he admitted to having a probable DVT some 6 years earlier with no obvious predisposing factors.

a. What differential diagnoses would you consider?
b. List four investigations that might aid his future management.

Data interpretation 15

A 6-year-old boy was seen by his family doctor. He had been febrile 10 days previously with rhinitis and a likely upper respiratory tract infection. On examination he appeared quite pale but with no other positive findings.

FBC showed:

Hb 5.2 g/dl
WBC $14.0 \times 10^9/l$
neutrophils $12.1 \times 10^9/l$
platelets $213 \times 10^9/l$

a. What differential diagnoses would you consider?
b. What further investigations would you arrange?

Data interpretation 16

A 48-year-old woman underwent elective hysterectomy for massive fibroids. The operation was entirely successful with no postoperative complications, although she was transfused 2 units of packed cells postoperatively. Seven days after surgery she was allowed home. Apart from paracetamol for pain she was receiving no regular medication. On the 10th postoperative day she phoned her GP because she had noticed widespread bruising over her legs and forearms.

A blood count was checked:

Hb 10.4 g/dl
MCV 83 fl
WBC 12.5 × 10⁹/l
platelets 4 × 10⁹/l

a. What is the likeliest cause of her current complication?
b. How would you confirm this?
c. Outline your management of this patient.

Data interpretation 17

A 21-year-old trainee bank clerk was noticed, by his work colleagues, to be rather plethoric. The patient's GP agreed with this observation but on direct questioning and physical examination he could find no abnormalities. He decided to check an FBC and biochemistry profile, which showed:

Hb 20.4 g/dl
RCC 6.21 × 10¹²/l
PCV 0.63
WBC 10.5 × 10⁹/l
platelets 416 × 10⁹/l

biochemistry screen – normal

a. What further investigations would you arrange?
b. What is your differential diagnosis?

Data interpretation 18

Figure 5.1 shows the results of a red cell investigation in which the percentage lysis of red cells is measured after exposing red blood cells to varying concentrations of saline.

a. What is the likely diagnosis?
b. What complications may arise from this disorder?
c. Describe the basic pathology of the disorder.

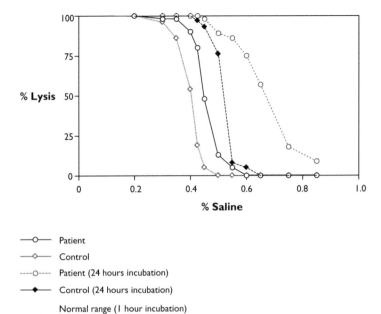

Fig. 5.1   Osmotic fragility test performed on patient's red cells and control red cells

Data interpretation 19

A 26-year-old woman gave birth to a healthy 7 lb (3.15 kg) baby girl. There were no complications during the pregnancy and labour was uneventful. This was her third child.

The day after delivery the staff noticed bruising on the baby's extremities and the paediatric team arranged to check an FBC and clotting screen on the baby which showed:

Hb 20.4 g/dl
RCC $6.0 \times 10^{12}/l$
MCV 100 fl
PCV 0.59
WBC $15.2 \times 10^9/l$
neutrophils $10 \times 10^9/l$
platelets $2 \times 10^9/l$

film comment: occasional nucleated red cell noted. Platelets on film agree with automated count

PT 13 s (normal range 12.0–14.0 s)
APTT 28.0 s (normal range 26.0–33.5 s)
fibrinogen 4.1 g/l (normal range 2.0–4.0 g/l)

a. What disorders may lead to these results?
b. How would you manage this neonate?

Data interpretation 20

An FBC from a 4-year-old boy with recurrent otitis media is shown below:

Hb 12.4 g/dl
WBC 1.6×10^9/l
neutrophils 0.2×10^9/l
platelets 284×10^9/l

a. Comment on the FBC results.
b. Name three causes for this abnormality.

Data interpretation 21

A 20-year-old music student presented with a 1-week history of lassitude, generalized aches and pains and had been noticed by her friends to be 'yellow'. Two weeks previously she also described an episode of sore throat and tender submandibular glands. Her past medical history was unremarkable. She was on no regular medication, although she took mefenamic acid occasionally for symptoms of dysmenorrhoea.

An FBC had been organized and showed:

Hb 7.7 g/dl
MCV 98 fl
MCHC 33.2 g/dl
MCH 31.8 pg
WBC 6.2×10^9/l
platelets 213×10^9/l

Urea, electrolytes and LFTs were also carried out with the following results:

serum sodium 141 mmol/l
serum potassium 3.7 mmol/l
serum bicarbonate 26 mmol/l
serum chloride 105 mmol/l
serum urea 3.0 mmol/l
serum creatinine 65 μmol/l
serum calcium 2.3 mmol/l
serum inorganic phosphate 1.3 mmol/l
serum total protein 69 g/l
serum bilirubin 47 μmol/l
serum alkaline phosphatase 96 i.u./l
serum aspartate transaminase 40 i.u./l

a. Specify four immediately helpful investigations.
b. What is the likely diagnosis?

Data interpretation 22

A 39-year-old woman developed severe postoperative bleeding following an elective tonsillectomy. Because of persistent bleeding, pallor and tachycardia a blood count and clotting were checked. These showed:

Hb 8.3 g/dl
MCV 82 fl
WBC 7.3 × 10^9/l
platelets 191 × 10^9/l

PT 44 s (normal 12.0–14.0 s)
APTT 83 s (normal 26.0–33.5 s)

She had previously been well apart from recurrent bouts of tonsillitis treated with antibiotics. She had two pregnancies; the youngest was 10 years old. A hysterectomy had been carried out 5 years previously because of menorrhagia. Postoperatively she had a DVT treated for 3 months with oral anticoagulants. Reviewing her casenotes showed her blood count, electrolytes and LFTs to have been normal some 6 weeks previously on samples taken at the outpatient clinic.

a. Suggest two likely causes for the abnormality.
b. What further investigation should be carried out to confirm the diagnosis?
c. Suggest appropriate immediate management.

Data interpretation 23

Mr S, a 52-year-old office worker, failed the finger prick test when he attended a blood donor session in his local church hall. He had been a regular donor for 15 years and never been shown to be anaemic. Over recent months he had noticed loose stools and mild weight loss, although his appetite was good and he ate a normal mixed diet. On examination he appeared well and of slim build; he had early finger clubbing. Investigations showed:

Hb 12.9 g/dl
MCV 113 fl
RCC 3.41 × 10^{12}/l
MCH 37.9 pg
WBC 8.5 × 10^9/l
neutrophils 6.2 × 10^9/l
platelets 554 × 10^9/l

film comment: anisocytosis, macrocytosis, a few hypochromic red cells; neutrophils show hypersegmentation

serum urea and electrolytes normal
serum calcium 2.03 mmol/l
serum bilirubin 24 μmol/l
serum vitamin B_{12} 90 ng/l (normal 150–700 ng/l)
red cell folate 92 μg/l (normal 150–700 μg/l)
serum ferritin 7 μg/l (normal range 15–300 μg/l)

a. What diagnosis or diagnoses would explain these findings?
b. What confirmatory tests would you arrange?
c. What complications are well recognized?

Data interpretation 24

A 55-year-old man presented to his family doctor with a 6-month history of worsening RA and weight loss. Before this period he had been in reasonably good health apart from controlled hypertension, for which he took captopril, and non-insulin-dependent diabetes mellitus. RA was diagnosed 15 years earlier and he required regular sulphasalazine. He had been admitted in the past with exacerbations of the disease which had been treated successfully on an inpatient basis.

He also complained of easy bruising and excessive bleeding following dental extraction performed 3 months earlier.

On examination he appeared reasonably well but with evidence of recent weight loss. Cardiovascular, respiratory and abdominal examinations were normal. Examination of his joints revealed obvious rheumatoid features but he did not have active synovitis. His GP arranged some coagulation tests that showed:

PT 12.3 s (normal range 12.0–14.0 s)
APTT 63 s (normal range 26.0–33.5 s)
fibrinogen 3.7 g/l (normal range 2.0–4.0 g/l)

APTT correction test (50:50 control: patient plasma) 52 s (normal range 26.0–33.5 s)

a. Comment on the results of the clotting studies.
b. What further test would you perform on the patient's plasma?

Data interpretation 25

A 32-year-old Asian woman consulted her GP since she had been feeling excessively tired. This had been progressive over the past several years but had been much worse over the past 3–4 months. She was finding that she had to rest during the day and was sleeping more than usual. She had four children aged 12, 11, 9 and 5 years. Her general health was good. Her appetite was normal and she ate a mixed diet. She complained of weight loss and felt she had lost around 4 kg in the last 6 months.

The GP examined her but found no abnormal physical findings. He arranged some blood tests:

Hb 9.9 g/dl
RCC 4.97 × 10^{12}/l
MCV 58.8 fl
WBC 7.3 × 10^9/l
neutrophils 4.4 × 10^9/l

blood film: pencil cells and target cells noted

serum vitamin B_{12} and red cell folate were normal
serum ferritin 54 μg/l (normal range 14–200 μg/l)

autoimmune profile normal apart from rheumatoid ELISA <10 i.u./l

viral screen – unremarkable
serum urea and electrolytes – normal
thyroid function tests – normal

a. Comment on the results shown above.
b. What further investigations would be useful?
c. How would you manage this patient?

Data interpretation 26

A 79-year-old retired army nurse presented with a 6-week history of night sweats, weight loss and discomfort on the left side of his abdomen. On examination gross splenomegaly with mild hepatomegaly were detected. There was no lymphadenopathy.
Investigations showed:

Hb 11.6 g/dl
WBC 72.5 × 10^9/l
platelets 123 × 10^9/l

film comment: lymphocytosis with many prolymphocytes

a. What further investigations would you perform?
b. What is the likely diagnosis?

Data interpretation 27

A 61-year-old woman presented during the winter months with a 10-week history of intermittent acrocyanosis involving the fingers of both hands. Examination revealed mild pallor and a tinge of jaundice. There was blue discoloration of both ear lobes and the spleen was palpable 3 cm below the left costal margin.

Investigations carried out were as follows:

Hb 9.8 g/dl
PCV 0.33
MCV 103.6 fl
MCH 47.1 pg
MCHC 46.2 g/dl
reticulocytes 4.5%
WBC $13.8 \times 10^9/l$
neutrophils $2.5 \times 10^9/l$
lymphocytes $10.1 \times 10^9/l$
monocytes $0.8 \times 10^9/l$
platelets $206 \times 10^9/l$

serum bilirubin 26 μmol/l

a. What is the probable cause of her symptoms?
b. What is the likely cause of the blood count anomalies and how might this be demonstrated?
c. What further investigations are indicated?
d. Discuss her further management.

Data interpretation 28

A 52-year-old woman was admitted as an emergency with pain and swelling in the left calf which had been present for 24 h. Investigation on admission confirmed the presence of a proximal femoral vein DVT. The patient had recently returned from holiday in New York and was in otherwise good health. Her past medical history consisted of one uncomplicated pregnancy 30 years before, appendicectomy 20 years before and DVT 15 years previously. She had also been anaemic in the past and had been treated with oral iron supplements. Her only other complaint was that she passed dark urine in the morning on occasions, but this was not a regular feature. Investigations on admission were as follows:

Hb 9.0 g/dl
MCV 76 fl
WBC 3.9 × 10^9/l
neutrophils 1.9 × 10^9/l
platelets 140 × 10^9/l
reticulocytes 8%

blood film comment: occasional polychromatic red cells noted; there are pencil cells and hypochromic red cells on the film

urea, electrolytes and LFTs – normal

On the basis of the above results her GP then requested haematinic assays.

a. What do you think the underlying diagnosis is in this case?
b. What further investigations would you perform?
c. Describe the underlying pathogenesis of this disorder.

Data interpretation 29

A 17-year-old youth presented to Accident and Emergency complaining of colicky abdominal pain which had been present for 3 h. He also described one episode of melaena. He gave a 2-day history of fever, polyarthralgia and the presence of a rash. In his past medical history he reported flu-like symptoms with an unproductive cough 3 or 4 weeks previously.

Clinically he had an urticarial rash with some haemorrhagic lesions over his buttocks and the extensor surfaces of the upper and lower limbs. He also had arthralgia of the knees, ankles, elbows and wrists but with no evidence of arthritis. His abdomen was diffusely tender with no guarding. Blood tests requested by the casualty officer revealed the following:

Hb 12.0 g/dl
WBC 17.0 × 10^9/l
platelets 210 × 10^9/l

clotting screen – normal

serum sodium 138 mmol/l
serum potassium 3.9 mmol/l
serum urea 8.0 mmol/l
serum creatinine 130 μmol/l

a. What further investigations would you perform?
b. What is the most likely diagnosis?
c. How would you manage this patient?

Data interpretation 30

A 67-year-old widow developed worsening dyspnoea, generalized fatigue, anorexia and worsening ankle oedema over a 2–3 month period. There had been no other specific symptoms. Her past medical history included an appendicectomy when she was 50. She had surgery carried out on a Dupuytren's contracture some 10 years previously. She was para 1+0. Some 6 years previously she had been seen and investigated for anaemia; she had had various blood tests, bone marrow tests and had received B_{12} supplementation for up to 2 years. She also had a long history of asthma for which she used salbutamol and beclomethasone inhalers regularly. She had been widowed 27 years previously.

She looked pale and had thin skin with several ecchymoses on both arms. There were some bruises on her lower limbs. Pulse was 82 beats/min and regular, BP 140/90 mmHg. Early Dupuytren's contractures were noted in both hands. There was some kyphosis and also hyperinflation of her chest consistent with past history of airways disease. Neurological examination was unremarkable. An FBC showed:

Hb 8.4 g/dl
MCV 128 fl
WBC $6.0 \times 10^9/l$
platelets $212 \times 10^9/l$
ESR 14 mm/1st hour (Westergren)

film comment: macrocytosis, some poikilocytes, occasional hypersegmented neutrophils identified

a. Specify a minimum of four differential diagnoses that you would consider.
b. Specify five further investigations you would initiate.

Data interpretation 31

A 52-year-old man presented complaining of increasing tiredness over the preceding 3 months. His medical history included a chole-cystectomy 10 years previously and a thoracotomy 3 years previously. He was a mild non-insulin-dependent diabetic managed with diet alone. His only medication was warfarin.

Examination revealed pallor and mild icterus. There were some fine inspiratory crepitations at the lung bases.

Investigations performed were as follows:

Hb 9.8 g/dl
PCV 0.34
MCV 76 fl
MCH 25 pg
MCHC 28 g/dl
reticulocytes 9%
WBC $11.0 \times 10^9/l$
neutrophils $7.3 \times 10^9/l$
lymphocytes $3.1 \times 10^9/l$
platelets $180 \times 10^9/l$

blood film: mild hypochromic features; a few schistocytes and spherocytes; normal platelet number and morphology

serum bilirubin 31 μmol/l

a. What is the likely diagnosis?
b. What further investigations are indicated?
c. What is the management?

Data interpretation 32

During a routine health check following a 3-week holiday to Thailand, a 35-year-old printer noticed a number of small bruises over his thighs and trunk. He denied any history of trauma but stated that he had had these for some months. His general health was good and he was taking no regular medication. He smoked 60 cigarettes per day and drank socially. His GP performed a blood count and clotting screen which showed:

Hb 16.3 g/dl
WBC $12.5 \times 10^9/l$
neutrophils $9.0 \times 10^9/l$
lymphocytes $2.1 \times 10^9/l$
platelets $118 \times 10^9/l$

PT 20 s (normal range 12.0–14.0 s)
APTT 46 s (26.0–33.5 s)
fibrinogen 3.2 g/l (normal range 2.0–4.0 g/l)

a. What further investigations would you consider in this patient?
b. What is the most likely diagnosis?

Data interpretation 33

A 7-year-old boy presented with a 3-day history of pains in the back and both legs. These had increased in severity over the previous 3 days and he was now unable to walk without stumbling.

Examination revealed pallor of the mucous membranes. There was generalized shotty (<1 cm) lymphadenopathy and the liver and spleen were both just palpable. He was exquisitely tender to palpation over both tibial tuberosities.

Investigations carried out were as follows:

Hb 7.9 g/dl
WBC 20.0 × 10^9/l
neutrophils 1.0 × 10^9/l
lymphocytes 5.0 × 10^9/l
monocytes 2.0 × 10^9/l
blast cells 12.0 × 10^9/l

blood film report: numerous monomorphic small blast cells with high nuclear : cytoplasmic ratio noted

CXR – normal

Monoclonal antibody	% positive cells
Anti-CD2	29%
Anti-CD3	28%
Anti-CD4	19%
Anti-CD10	59%
Anti-CD19	55%
Anti-HLA DR (class II)	61%
Anti-surface immunoglobulin	3%

Membrane phenotype of peripheral blood mononuclear cells (determined by indirect immunofluorescence):

a. What is the diagnosis?
b. What further investigations would you perform?
c. What features may influence the prognosis?

Data interpretation 34

A 36-year-old woman was admitted to hospital with suspected DVT of the left leg. Venography was carried out and this confirmed the clinical suspicions and showed proximal venous thrombosis.

From the history elicited by the house physician, the patient had a DVT some 15 years earlier and suspected DVT 10 years subsequently, although this was never confirmed radiologically. The patient was taking no regular medication other than the combined oral contraceptive pill. There was no family history of note.

The house physician ordered a few baseline investigations, the results of which showed:

Hb 13.2 g/dl
MCV 79 fl
WBC 7.3 × 10^9/l
platelets 189 × 10^9/l

PT 13 s (normal range 12.0–14.0 s)
APTT 56 s (normal range 26.0–33.5 s)
fibrinogen 3.5 g/l (normal range 2.0–4.0 g/l)

a. What further investigations should be performed in this patient?
b. Briefly discuss the management.

Data interpretation 35

A 55-year-old woman with known long-standing follicular NHL was seen urgently in outpatients following deterioration of her condition.

She had originally presented 2 years previously with asymptomatic generalized adenopathy. A lymph node biopsy showed follicular lymphoma of low-grade type and she was treated with chlorambucil at a dose of 10 mg daily for 14 days out of each 28 days for 4 months. Four months prior to her present referral she had noticed a recurrence of generalized adenopathy. She was otherwise asymptomatic and her glands were of low volume. Therefore no action was taken.

On this occasion she had noticed sudden onset of thirst and abdominal distension with associated increasing back pain and night sweats.

On examination, low-volume adenopathy was present as previously described and was unchanged. She did, however, have tense ascites. Her FBC showed:

Hb 9.6 g/dl
WBC $2.9 \times 10^9/l$
platelets $48 \times 10^9/l$

serum urea 6.2 mmol/l
serum creatinine 76 μmol/l
serum potassium 4.5 mmol/l
serum calcium 3.2 mmol/l
serum albumin 28 g/l
serum bilirubin 4 μmol/l

a. What is the likely diagnosis?
b. Name three diagnostic tests, ranked in order of importance, that would help determine her future treatment.

Data interpretation 36

A 4-year-old Asian boy was referred for investigation of anaemia. His parents had noticed that he looked pale but he had no other symptoms and had been developing normally.

Investigations performed at that time were as follows:

Hb 6.6 g/dl
RCC $5.5 \times 10^{12}/l$
MCV 59 fl
WBC $6.8 \times 10^9/l$
neutrophils $3.8 \times 10^9/l$
lymphocytes $2.2 \times 10^9/l$
platelets $264 \times 10^9/l$

blood film examination: hypochromic microcytic red cells, target cells, occasional nucleated red blood cells

haemoglobin electrophoresis: HbA_2 2%
                                 HbF   98%

Over the next 5 years, he developed moderate (5 cm) splenomegaly and required blood transfusion on six occasions. He grew normally and had minimal symptoms.

a. What is the likely diagnosis?
b. Comment on the pathogenesis of this condition.
c. What is the management?

Data interpretation 37

An 18-year-old previously fit man presented to the outpatients department with a 4–6-week history of increasing cough with associated dyspnoea and facial swelling. During this period of time he had lost 7 kg in weight and had felt extremely tired. He was employed as an electrical fitter and admitted to smoking 20 cigarettes daily. His hobbies included weight lifting.

On examination he appeared short of breath on minimal exertion. His chest wall was displaced anteriorly and superior vena caval obstruction was apparent. Abdominal examination was normal.

A CXR showed a large anterior mediastinal mass with bilateral small-volume pleural effusions.

a. Give three diagnostic possibilities accounting for these features.
b. How would you investigate this man?

Data interpretation 38

A 24-h full-term infant was found to be jaundiced. A full serological screen on the infant and parents showed the following results:

ABO grouping

	Red cells tested with			Serum tested with	
	Anti-A	Anti-B	Anti-A,B	A cells	B cells
Father	5+	0	5+	0	4+
Mother	0	0	0	5+	5+
Infant	5+	0	5+		

Rhesus D typing

	Anti-D	Anti-D	AB serum
Father	5+	5+	0
Mother	0	0	0
Infant	5+	5+	0

DCT on infant cells

Polyspecific AHG: 4+

Antibody screening of the maternal serum is demonstrated in Fig. 5.2:

Name	ABO	Rh type	M	N	S	s	P_1	Lu a	Lu b	Le a	Le b	K	k	Kp^aKp^b		Fy a	Fy b	Jk a	Jk b	Enzyme papain	Saline 16°C	Saline 37°C	IAGT
1	0	R_1R_1	0	+	0	+	0	+	+	0	+	+	+	+	0	+	+	+	+	4+	0	0	4+
2	0	R_2R_2	+	+	+	0	+	0	+	0	+	0	+	0	+	+	0	0	+	5+	0	0	4+
3	0	R_1r	+	0	+	+	+	0	+	0	0	+	+	0	+	0	+	+	+	4+	0	0	4+
4	0	rr	+	+	+	+	+	+	+	0	+	+	+	0	+	+	0	0	+	0	0	0	0
5	0	rr	0	+	0	+	0	0	+	0	+	0	+	0	+	+	+	+	0	0	0	0	0
6	0	rr	+	0	+	+	+	0	+	+	0	0	+	0	+	0	+	+	0	4+	2+	2+	3+
7	0	r'r	+	0	+	0	+	0	+	+	0	0	+	+	+	0	+	0	+	4+	1+	3+	4+
8	0	r"r	+	+	+	+	+	0	+	0	0	0	+	0	+	+	+	+	+	0	0	0	0
patient's own																					0	0	0

Fig. 5.2   Maternal serum tested against panel of typed red cells

a. What are the blood groups of mother, father and infant?
b. What may be the cause of the baby's jaundice?
c. What should be the group of any blood transfused to the baby?

Data interpretation 39

Six days after an apparently uneventful blood transfusion post-partum, a multiparous woman appeared unduly jaundiced and developed oliguria. She remained somewhat anaemic. The following were her serological findings:

ABO grouping

	Patient and donor red cells tested with specific antisera			Patient's serum tested with known A and B cells	
	Anti-A	Anti-B	Anti-A,B	A cells	B cells
Pre-transfusion sample	0	0	0	4+	4+
Post-transfusion sample	0	0	0	5+	4+
Donation 1	0	0	0		
Donation 2	0	0	0		
Donation 3	0	0	0		

Rhesus D typing

	Patient and donor red cells tested with specific antisera		
	Anti-D	Anti-D	AB serum
Pre-transfusion sample	0	0	0
Post-transfusion sample	0	0	0
Donation 1	0	0	0
Donation 2	0	0	0
Donation 3	0	0	0

DCT

	Polyspecific AHG
Pre-transfusion sample	0
Post-transfusion sample	1+ (mixed field)

Cross-matching

Pre-transfusion sample

Donation number	Immediate spin	Agglutination 37°C	IAGT
Donation 1	0	0	0
Donation 2	0	0	0
Donation 3	0	0	0

Post-transfusion sample

Donation number	Immediate spin	Agglutination 37°C	IAGT
Donation 1	0	0	0
Donation 2	0	0	3+
Donation 3	0	0	3+

Figs 5.3 and 5.4 show results of antibody screening of the pre- and post-transfusion samples

Name	ABO	Rh type	M	N	S	s	P1	Lu a	Lu b	Le a	Le b	K	k	Kp^a	Kp^b	Fy a	Fy b	Jk a	Jk b	Enzyme papain	Saline 16°C	Saline 37°C	IAGT
1	0	R_1R_1	0	+	0	+	0	+	+	0	+	+	+	+	0	+	+	+	+	5+	0	3+	5+
2	0	R_2R_2	+	+	+	0	+	0	+	0	+	0	+	0	+	+	0	0	+	5+	0	4+	5+
3	0	R_1r	+	0	+	+	+	0	+	0	0	+	+	0	+	0	+	+	+	5+	0	3+	4+
4	0	rr	+	+	+	+	+	+	+	0	+	+	+	0	+	+	0	0	+	0	0	0	0
5	0	rr	0	+	0	+	0	0	+	0	+	0	+	0	+	+	+	+	0	0	0	0	0
6	0	rr	+	0	+	+	+	0	+	+	0	0	+	0	+	0	+	+	0	0	0	0	0
7	0	r'r	+	0	+	0	+	0	+	+	0	0	+	+	+	0	+	0	+	0	0	0	0
8	0	r"r	+	+	+	+	+	0	+	0	0	0	+	0	+	+	+	+	+	0	0	0	0
patient's own																				0	0	0	0

Fig. 5.3   Pre-transfusion sample

Name	ABO	Rh type	M	N	S	s	P1	Lu a	Lu b	Le a	Le b	K	k	Kp^a	Kp^b	Fy a	Fy b	Jk a	Jk b	Enzyme papain	Saline 16°C	Saline 37°C	IAGT
1	0	R_1R_1	0	+	0	+	0	+	+	0	+	+	+	+	0	+	+	+	+	5+	0	4+	4+
2	0	R_2R_2	+	+	+	0	+	0	+	0	+	0	+	0	+	+	0	0	+	5+	0	4+	5+
3	0	R_1r	+	0	+	+	+	0	+	0	0	+	+	0	+	0	+	+	+	5+	0	3+	4+
4	0	rr	+	+	+	+	+	+	+	0	+	+	+	0	+	+	0	0	+	0	0	0	0
5	0	rr	0	+	0	+	0	0	+	0	+	0	+	0	+	+	+	+	0	2+	0	0	3+
6	0	rr	+	0	+	+	+	0	+	+	0	0	+	0	+	0	+	+	0	2+	0	0	3+
7	0	r'r	+	0	+	0	+	0	+	+	0	0	+	+	+	0	+	0	+	0	0	0	0
8	0	r"r	+	+	+	+	+	0	+	0	0	0	+	0	+	+	+	+	+	2+	0	0	2+
patient's own																				0	0	0	1+

Fig. 5.4   Post-transfusion sample

a. How would you interpret the serological data?
b. What blood would you select for transfusion?

Data interpretation 40

A 76-year-old woman was admitted to hospital with a severe lower respiratory tract infection requiring intravenous antibiotics. An FBC, urea and electrolytes were checked on admission and these showed:

Hb 9.8 g/dl
MCV 58 fl
WBC $17.0 \times 10^9/l$
neutrophils $13.4 \times 10^9/l$
platelets $86 \times 10^9/l$

blood film: microcytic hypochromic red cells; there is prominent basophilic stippling; target cells and teardrop red cells are noted

serum urea and electrolytes – normal

a. Comment on the FBC indices.
b. On reviewing her casenotes it was found that an FBC checked 3 years previously was normal. What further investigations would you arrange?

6 | Answers to data interpretation questions

Data interpretation 1

a. Peripheral blood film examination.
Paul–Bunnell or Monospot test for glandular fever.
Viral serology for EBV, CMV and toxoplasmosis.
Peripheral blood cell markers to differentiate an infective from leukaemic cause for the lymphocytosis.
Bone marrow aspirate and trephine to exclude underlying haematological disease such as lymphoma or leukaemia.
CT chest and abdomen for lymphadenopathy.
b. The diagnosis in this case was EBV infection (infectious mononucleosis; glandular fever) but would fit clinically with CMV or toxoplasma infection.

Glandular fever often presents non-specifically but may produce dramatic physical findings and a bizarre blood film that may resemble an acute leukaemia. The diagnosis can usually be made from the history, blood film and Monospot test alone. However, there are occasions when a bone marrow is performed to exclude leukaemia if the morphology is grossly abnormal and viral screens prove negative.

> The 'mononucleosis syndromes' are the commonest cause of benign lymphocytosis. EBV and CMV are the commonest causes. EBV results in heterophile-antibody-positive and CMV heterophile-antibody-negative illnesses. Lymphadenopathy is a feature of EBV rather than CMV infection; in both cases the atypical lymphocytes are T cells.
>
> EBV is transmitted via saliva whilst CMV is spread by sexual contact or breast milk as well as droplet spread. EBV attaches to and infects B cells in tonsils via complement surface receptors. B cell stimulation occurs and generates a response in T cells against infected B cells. This results in the characteristic pharyngitis and circulating atypical lymphocytes.

Final diagnosis

Infectious mononucleosis.

Data interpretation 2

a. An acute-onset haemolytic anaemia.
b. Reticulocyte count.
   DAT (DCT).
   LFTs, including bilirubin.
   Urinalysis for urobilinogen, haemosiderin, haemoglobin, etc.
   Serum haptoglobins for evidence of recent haemolysis.
   A detailed further history for ingestion of/exposure to drugs, toxins, etc.

The reticulocytes were raised at 9%; DAT was negative. Bilirubin was elevated at 46 μmol/l; urinalysis showed haemoglobinuria and urinary urobilinogen; haptoglobins were absent. These features together with the clinical picture suggest ongoing haemolysis, i.e. reduced red cell lifespan due to increased destruction.

A repeat FBC 24 h after admission showed a further fall in Hb to 6.8 g/dl. The film showed increased numbers of fragmented cells with a characteristic 'bite cell' morphology. The clinical features were thus strongly suggestive of oxidative haemolysis and further history-taking revealed that the individual had eaten large numbers of raw beans a few days prior to presentation. He was managed supportively with a 2-unit packed red cell transfusion and oral folic acid. The haemolytic episode settled within 3–5 days. Follow-up testing showed him to have G6PD deficiency.

> Most commonly, an acute presentation of anaemia reflects bleeding; the absence of a clear history of blood loss and the history of rigors were suggestive of acquired haemolysis in this case. The negative antiglobulin test rapidly identified a likely non-immune cause for the anaemia; the film changes and rapid onset were suspicious of acute oxidative haemolysis, in this case due to favism. G6PD deficiency does occur in northern Europeans and would more typically result from drug therapy with dapsone, sulphasalazine or chloroquine. Confirmation of deficiency should be done after haemolysis has settled, has enzyme levels are higher in reticulocytes. Acute episodes are managed supportively.

Final diagnosis

Acute haemolysis secondary to G6PD deficiency (favism).

Data interpretation 3

a. Bleeding time.
   Mixing studies or correction tests (i.e. addition of normal plasma to the patient's plasma in 50 : 50 mix to determine whether the abnormal clotting results are due to deficiency of a coagulation factor or to the presence of an inhibitor).
   vWF:Ag concentration.
   RiCoF assay.
   Anticardiolipin (lupus) antibody.
b. von Willebrand's disease.

The bleeding time in this patient was 15 min (normal 3–9 min). The addition of normal plasma corrected the abnormal APTT. This patient's vWF:Ag and RiCoF were reduced suggesting a diagnosis of von Willebrand's disease, an autosomal dominant disorder of coagulation which also affects platelet function. Patients suffer from mucosal and soft-tissue bleeding typically following dental extraction or minor surgery. Treatment consists of desmopressin (DDAVP), intermediate-purity FVIII concentrate and, in life-threatening bleeds, cryoprecipitate. Cryoprecipitate is used infrequently now due to risk of transmission of viral infection, including HIV and hepatitis C.

> von Willebrand factor is a protein involved in platelet adhesion to subendothelium, and plays an active role in platelet aggregation. The molecule also acts as a carrier for the large FVIII molecule (protective effect). von Willebrand factor is synthesized in platelets and endothelial cells in blood vessels; the gene is located on chromosome 12. The molecules form multimers in plasma and may be estimated using either ELISA techniques or Laurell rockets. The Laurell rockets have now been replaced in most haematology departments by the ELISA method.
>
> RiCoF represents the activity of plasma von Willebrand factor in promoting the aggregation of washed platelets in conjunction with the antibiotic ristocetin. Ristocetin induces platelet aggregation through the glycoprotein molecules on platelet membranes.
>
> Multimer analysis is performed by electrophoresis and staining using anti-von Willebrand factor antibodies.
>
> There are several types of von Willebrand's disease (e.g. I, IIa, IIb, III, platelet type and Normandy variant). Type I constitutes 70% of cases and results from the production of a structurally normal von Willebrand factor protein but present in reduced amount. Consequently vWF:Ag, RiCoF and VIII:C are reduced but with normal multimeric pattern on electrophoresis. The inheritance is autosomal dominant.
>
> Type II von Willebrand's disease makes up 20% of cases. Again, inheritance is autosomal dominant. In this subtype there is a structural abnormality in von Willebrand's factor leading to failure of production of high-molecular-weight multimers. The von Willebrand's factor antigen may be relatively spared compared with RiCoF, which is reduced.

Classification of von Willebrand's disease

Type	Inheritance	VIII:C	vWF:Ag	RiCoF	Multimer analysis
I	Autosomal dominant	L	L	L	Normal pattern
IIa	Autosomal dominant	L or N	L or N	L	Large and intermediate multimers absent from plasma and platelets, abnormal triplets
IIb	Autosomal dominant	L or N	L or N	L or N	Large multimers absent from plasma only, normal triplets
IIc	Autosomal recessive	N	N	L	Large multimers absent from plasma and platelets, abnormal triplets
III	Autosomal recessive	L	L	0	None detected

L: low; N: normal; 0: absent.

Bleeding in von Willebrand's disease is predominantly mucosal with nose bleeds, bruising, heavy periods, gum bleeding and bleeding after dental extraction. Bleeding into joints and muscles is not a feature of von Willebrand's disease.

The management is aimed at correcting the VIII:C abnormality using, for example, desmopressin (DDAVP). This increases VIII:C and RiCoF three to five times the basal level due to release of stored von Willebrand's factor from endothelial cells. This is recommended for patients with mild to moderate von Willebrand's disease undergoing moderate haemostatic stress (e.g. minor operation). The effect of DDAVP lasts 4–8 h. It is useful in type I von Willebrand's disease but is not recommended in type IIb (platelet aggregation); the dosage used is 0.3–0.4 μg/kg i.v. 12-hourly. Alternatively, intermediate-purity FVIII concentrate may be used since this contains von Willebrand's factor multimers (high-purity FVIII does not).

Cryoprecipitate, the previous mainstay of treatment, is used little now due to the infection risk associated with this blood product.

Final diagnosis

von Willebrand's disease type I.

Data interpretation 4

a. These indices are those of a hypochromic microcytic anaemia and the main differential diagnoses are iron-deficiency anaemia and thalassaemia.
b. Serum ferritin estimation.
   Serum iron/TIBC.
   Hb A$_2$ estimation.
   Hb electrophoresis.
   Full clinical history, including menstrual history and other pointers to overt and occult blood loss, should be obtained e.g. FOBs.
   Full family history should be sought.

This patient had simple iron-deficiency anaemia and her serum ferritin was <4 μg/l (normal range 14–200 μg/l). The serum iron was 5 μmol/l (normal range 11–28 μmol/l) and TIBC was 90 μmol/l (normal range 45–75 μmol/l) consistent with this diagnosis. Thalassaemia is an inherited disorder of globin synthesis which may cause a microcytic anaemia in the absence of iron deficiency. In β-thalassaemia HbA$_2$ ($\alpha_2\delta_2$) is elevated.

In addition to the investigations listed above it is mandatory to take a full clinical history, including menstrual history. Other pointers to overt and occult blood loss should be sought. Obtaining a detailed family history is important in the evaluation of anaemias, especially when thalassaemia is being considered.

Final diagnosis

Iron-deficiency anaemia secondary to menorrhagia ± adolescent growth spurt.

Data interpretation 5

a. Haematinic assays (serum vitamin B$_{12}$/folate/ferritin).
   Bone marrow aspirate and trephine biopsy.
   CXR.
b. MDS.
   Marrow infiltration secondary to haematological malignancy or other cancer (e.g. bowel, lung, prostate).

This patient had MDS, a pre-leukaemic disorder in some cases. It is commoner in older patients and may result in pancytopenia, as in this case. The platelets are reduced and are functionally abnormal; hence bleeding is common, even when the platelet count is reasonably high (cf. ITP where bleeding is not common until the platelet count drops below $15 \times 10^9/l$). Treatment is supportive, with red cell and platelet transfusions. Antibiotics are sometimes given prophylactically to reduce the incidence of infection. In many cases the disease will progress to acute leukaemia, most often myeloid in type.

Haematinic assays are performed to exclude pancytopenia secondary to, for example, vitamin B_{12} deficiency. In cases where pancytopenia is due to bone marrow infiltration by disseminated carcinoma or leukaemia/lymphoma, bone marrow aspirate and trephine biopsy are helpful.

Final diagnosis

Myelodysplastic syndrome.

Data interpretation 6

a. The clinical presentation and clotting abnormality indicate a likely disorder of the intrinsic clotting pathway. Haemophilia A (FVIII deficiency) or Haemophilia B (FIX deficiency. Christmas disease) are the commonest and by far the most likely in a male patient. Laboratory testing is needed to distinguish between the two. von Willebrand's disease is also a possibility. Clinical features are similar; milder cases may be asymptomatic until they face a significant haemostatic challenge such as surgery.
b. Further investigations should include:
   (i)   Correction experiments mixing 50% normal plasma in the APTT test, which would show improvement and therefore indicate a factor deficiency.
   (ii) Measuring the bleeding time, which would be normal in either type of haemophilia and therefore differentiate from von Willebrand's disease.
   (iii) Assaying clotting factors VIII and IX. Figure 6.1 shows an APTT-based FIX assay of reference (100% FIX) and patient plasma. Samples were tested undiluted (100%), at $1:3$ (33%) and $1:9$ dilution (11.1%). This assay tests the ability of patient plasma to correct the prolonged APTT of a substrate (FIX deficient) plasma. Patient and reference plasmas are added to substrate plasma and an APTT

performed. Drawing a horizontal line from the 100% point on the patient's plasma and dropping a perpendicular determines the patient's factor level.

This patient was found to have Christmas disease with low levels of FIX on assay.

Other factors to be considered in the differential include heparin administration and – much less likely – liver disease. In a patient presenting with FIX deficiency the absence of a family history is not unusual; a percentage of cases present as new mutations.

Immediate management combines local measures and transfusion of fresh frozen plasma until the defect is classified as FVIII or FIX deficiency, since different factor products are required for each condition.

Final diagnosis

Haemophilia B (FIX deficiency).

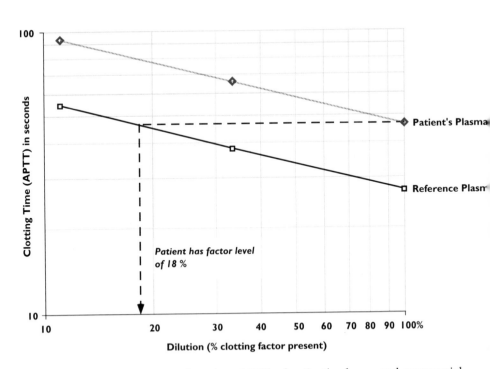

Fig. 6.1 Factor IX assay (based on APTT) of patient's plasma and commercial reference plasma (FIX level 100%) used to determine FIX level in patient plasma

Data interpretation 7

a. Chronic bleeding is the result of a low plasma fibrinogen (as measured by a functional assay).
b. Iron-deficiency anaemia.
c. Fibrinogen should be assayed by a chemical and immunological method to distinguish hypofibrinogenaemia from dysfibrinogenaemia.
d. The iron-deficient state should be treated with oral iron replacement. In hereditary disorders of fibrinogen, the need for replacement therapy is determined from the clinical picture and past medical history. Generally, patients with severe haemorrhage or those undergoing surgical procedures need replacement and cryoprecipitate is the most practical source of fibrinogen. Antifibrinolytic agents may be helpful in less severe bleeding, as in this patient.

This patient suffered from hereditary dysfibrinogenaemia. The prolonged thrombin time points to a defect in the function and/or amount of fibrinogen and the prolonged reptilase time excludes a heparin effect as the cause of the coagulation test abnormalities. The fibrinogen level is reduced by the functional (Clauss) assay, but both the chemical and immunological estimations were in the normal range, thus demonstrating a normal amount of functionally defective fibrinogen.

Hereditary dysfibrinogenaemias need to be distinguished from hereditary afibrinogenaemia (and hypofibrinogenaemia) where functional, chemical and immunological assays of fibrinogen are reduced in parallel. The dysfibrinogenaemias are a heterogeneous group of disorders. Inheritance is autosomal dominant in the majority of cases, but a positive family history is often lacking, presumably reflecting new mutations or clinical variability. More than 200 variants are described and include defects of fibrinopeptide release, polymerization defects and defects of stabilization. Over half of all hereditary dysfibrinogenaemia patients are asymptomatic. Abnormal bleeding occurs in approximately one-third while, paradoxically, thrombotic manifestations are seen in the remaining one-sixth.

Dysfibrinogenaemia may be seen as an acquired disorder in a number of clinical settings, including liver disease, acute pancreatitis and in association with malignancies (hepatoma, renal cell carcinoma and lymphoma).

Final diagnosis

Dysfibrinogenaemia.

Data interpretation 8

a. Folate deficiency secondary to alcohol abuse.
b. Haematinic assays including serum vitamin B_{12}, serum folate and serum ferritin.
   Blood alcohol level.
c. Immediate supportive care of the unconscious patient, including airway, breathing and circulation.
   Abstention from alcohol.
   Folate replacement.

This man was found to have acute folate deficiency secondary to prolonged and excessive alcohol abuse. The haematological indices along with the blood film features are highly suggestive of a haematinic deficiency and assays performed confirmed this diagnosis. The management consists of removal of the offending agent which, in this case, was alcohol, and folic acid supplementation. Alcoholics may become deficient in folate due to a poor diet. The film features could equally have been due to vitamin B_{12} deficiency which produces an identical haematological profile and blood film. In cases such as these, subdural haematoma should always be considered and a CT scan performed if clinically indicated.

Final diagnosis

Severe folate deficiency.

Data interpretation 9

a. Marrow infiltration (carcinoma, primary haematological disease, e.g. myeloma, leukaemia, myeloproliferative disease, lymphoma).
   Causes of secondary reactive changes such as haemorrhage, inflammation, infection, etc.
b. ESR.
   Bone marrow aspirate and trephine biopsy.
   Serum immunoglobulins and protein electrophoresis.
   Full biochemistry screen including bone and renal profile.
   Serum calcium level.
   Autoantibody screen.
   CXR.

The platelet count may be elevated in response to haemorrhage, infection, etc. However, the platelet count is not commonly raised above $1000 \times 10^9/l$ as a 'reactive' phenomenon. The presence of rouleaux and myelocytes in the peripheral blood film in this patient, along with the grossly elevated platelet count, is highly suggestive of underlying neoplastic disease. This includes haematological malignancies as well as non-haematological neoplasms such as secondary carcinomas (e.g. breast, lung, prostate, bowel, thyroid).

Final diagnosis

Reactive thrombocytosis secondary to underlying breast carcinoma.

Data interpretation 10

a. The features are suggestive of a mild sickle crisis.
b. She clearly has HbS as determined by Hb electrophoresis. She also has some HbA ($\alpha_2\beta_2$) indicative of the presence of some normal β-globin (it should be absent if she has homozygous sickle cell disease, HbS containing β^s). She also has elevation of HbA$_2$ ($\alpha_2\delta_2$) which is characteristic of β-thalassaemia trait. Therefore, she has sickle/β^+-thalassaemia (had she been sickle/β^0-thalassaemia, there would have been no HbA). Investigation of her parents showed her mother had sickle cell trait (AS) and her father had β^+-thalassaemia trait.
c. Unlike straightforward sickle trait, sickle/thalassaemia patients suffer crises and need to be managed in the standard manner. On admission, patients should be examined for signs of infection. Intravenous fluids, oxygen and analgesia should be commenced along with i.v. or oral broad-spectrum antibiotics (e.g. ampicillin). An FBC, urea and electrolytes, CXR, MSU and blood cultures should be checked. With the above measures the crisis will usually subside within a few days.

　　For the longer term, the patient should be given a haemoglobinopathy card advising other clinicians of her genotype; she should be counselled by a trained haemoglobinopathy counsellor, and be prescribed folic acid (remember that low-grade ongoing haemolysis is a feature) and a week's supply of antibiotics for use when a crisis is suspected. Patients should also be warned about the precipitants of crises, e.g. dehydration, excessive cold, etc.

le cell disease is the result of inheritance of homozygous β^s, a point mutation in the sixth amino acid of the β-globin chain which substitutes glu→val. This form of haemoglobin polymerizes at reduced oxygen tension, leading to sickling of red cells that are less deformable and this leads to vaso-occlusive disease. Red cells have decreased survival. Haemolysis leads to chronic anaemia, jaundice, increased cardiac output, delayed growth in children, predisposition to gallstones and anaemic crises. The occlusion of the microvasculature leads to tissue ischaemia and pain. Other vaso-occlusive complications include priapism, stroke, liver and renal impairment, aseptic necrosis of the femur, leg ulcers and proliferative retinopathy.

> As well as HbSS (sickle cell disease), there are a number of other disorders with features similar to HbSS, such as in this case. These include sickle/β-thalassaemia, HbSC (i.e. HbS and HbC). Other disorders such as HbSD and HbS/α-thalassaemia are milder than HbSS but more severe than sickle trait.

Final diagnosis

Sickle/β^+-thalassaemia.

Data interpretation 11

a. Clotting factor deficiency rather than inhibitor, since the APTT normalizes after normal control plasma is added to the patient's plasma. The APTT also becomes normal when the patient's plasma is mixed with adsorbed plasma (lacking factors II, VII, IX and X) but does not correct on the addition of aged serum (lacking factors I, II, V, VIII). The likeliest deficiency is FVIII.
b. FVIII assay. This confirmed reduction in the patient's FVIII level to ~19% (normal range 50–150%).
c. Oral tranexamic acid may be used to help control bleeding. For severe bleeding episodes, i.v. FVIII may be used to bring the patient's FVIII level up sufficiently to control bleeding. Similarly, to cover dental extractions or other procedures likely to cause bleeding, prophylactic FVIII should be given. At 19% the patient should not require regular FVIII since the deficiency is relatively mild.

Final diagnosis

Mild haemophilia A (FVIII deficiency).

Data interpretation 12

a. Cell surface markers (immunophenotype).
    Serum immunoglobulin quantitation.
    CXR.
    Abdominal ultrasound.
    CT of the abdomen and chest.
    Bone marrow aspirate and trephine biopsy.
    Examination of the optic fundi.
b. Waldenström's macroglobulinaemia.
    This is a low-grade NHL characterized by IgM paraprotein
    production. This patient was found to have an IgM of 74 g/l
    and immunophenotype confirmed the presence of a mono-
    clonal B cell population expressing IgM κ.
    CXR revealed mild cardiac enlargement.
    Splenomegaly was confirmed on the abdominal ultrasound.
    The marrow aspirate confirmed the lymphocytosis and
    trephine biopsy showed lymphoid infiltration.
    Examination of the fundi confirmed grossly distended blood
    vessels and numerous haemorrhages consistent with a clinical
    diagnosis of hyperviscosity syndrome.
c. The basic management principles are:
    (i)   to confirm the diagnosis (as above);
    (ii)   to reduce the patient's plasma viscosity manually by
           exchange transfusion or plasma exchange (cell separator);
    (iii) adequate hydration and introduction of chemotherapy –
           chlorambucil or fludarabine would be likely drugs;
    (iv)   transfusion of red cells is not recommended (hypervis-
           cosity) but, if absolutely essential, should be given slowly
           and preferably over 2 days.

Final diagnosis

**Low-grade lymphoma with associated IgM paraproteinaemia
(Waldenström's macroglobulinaemia).**

Data interpretation 13

a. Essential (primary) thrombocythaemia (ET).
Secondary thrombocythaemia, e.g. malignant disease.
Chronic inflammation.
Acute inflammation.
Acute blood loss.
Postoperatively, especially post-splenectomy.
Prematurity.
b. Since the platelets exceed $1000 \times 10^9/l$ and other causes are not obvious then ET is likeliest.
c. The patient needs to be screened for secondary causes (CXR, occult malignancy search, autoimmune profile, infection screen, etc.). A bone marrow and trephine biopsy should be performed in order to determine whether the thrombocythaemia is primary or secondary, although this is not a diagnostic test in the true sense.
d. If thrombotic and/or bleeding complications are present, consider urgent platelet reduction using plateletpheresis. Otherwise oral hydroxyurea should be used to reduce the platelet count over days to weeks.

ET is one of the myeloproliferative disorders and typically affects people between 50 and 70 years of age; males and females are equally affected. Diagnosis may be made on routine blood testing and many patients have few symptoms. Abdominal examination is usually normal but may reveal mild splenomegaly in a proportion of cases (40%). Mitral and aortic valve thickening have been reported in a few patients but the aetiology of this is unknown. Although the platelet count is high, bleeding, as well as thrombosis, is a major risk. Patients may complain of burning discomfort in their hands or feet (erythromelalgia) and this may be confused with Raynaud's phenomenon.

The blood count shows a grossly elevated platelet count. There may be mild elevation of WBC and mild anaemia. The blood film, as well as showing a high platelet count, may also show large platelets.

Bone marrow trephine biopsy may show increased numbers of megakaryocytes (from which platelets are derived) and clustering of megakaryocytes highly suggestive of ET. Increased ploidy of megakaryocytes on trephine biopsy is a further feature of ET.

No single test can diagnose ET with complete confidence and, in part, it is a diagnosis of exclusion.

> Treatment is aimed at reducing the platelet count to a safe level, although there is no firm evidence to suggest that the prognosis is improved with chronic platelet-reducing therapy. Hydroxyurea is a myelosuppressive (non-alkylating) agent that is highly effective in ET and patients generally require 10–30 mg/kg per day. Other treatments include busulphan, interferon-α and ^{32}P. Antiplatelet drugs (e.g. aspirin) may be of value in patients with thrombotic complications. A new agent, anagrelide, is not routinely available in the UK but it is commonly used for this condition in the USA. The reasons for treatment are to reduce the incidence of bleeding and thrombotic complications. Both are a risk of this condition when the platelet count is markedly increased. Low-dose aspirin therapy would also be recommended, although this should be avoided where cases have predominantly haemorrhagic manifestations. With normalization of platelet count, haemorrhagic and thrombotic risks are greatly reduced.

The mildly elevated serum calcium and albumin were probably due to venous stasis whilst the samples were being taken. Repeat sampling without using a tourniquet was normal.

Final diagnosis

Myeloproliferative disease; ET.

Data interpretation 14

a. This is a young man with recurrent thromboembolic disease (thrombophilia). Underlying disorders might include:
Protein C deficiency.
Protein S deficiency.
Antithrombin III deficiency.
Lupus anticoagulant.
APCR.

b. Thrombophilia screening (i.e. protein C, S, etc. levels) is not of value in the acute event since coagulation factors are used up in the thrombotic process and patients are generally anticoagulated. Instead, investigation should be carried out when the patient is off anticoagulants since warfarin, for example, depletes vitamin K-dependent clotting factors (factors II, VII, IX and X as well as proteins C and S).

> It is worth checking a coagulation screen including tests for lupus anticoagulant. Other investigations should include autoimmune profile, protein C, S and antithrombin III (off anticoagulants) and APCR. APCR testing is carried out by a clotting test and, more recently, a PCR method which detects a point mutation in the factor V gene (factor V Leiden mutation) that predisposes to APCR and thrombophilia. The Leiden mutation is the same in every case and a single set of PCR primers generates an amplified fragment of DNA that is digested with Mnl I

restriction enzyme. Normal subjects show a characteristic DNA fragment size after restriction digestion that is quite different to the heterozygote with the factor V Leiden mutation. This method of PCR amplification followed by restriction digestion is analogous to that used for diagnosis of sickle cell disease.

APCR is inherited in an autosomal dominant fashion and may be the most common inherited thrombophilia. It has been shown that patients with both protein C deficiency and the factor V Leiden mutation are at increased risk of thromboembolic disease.

Acquired hypercoagulable states include:

Venous stasis.
Malignancy.
Lupus anticoagulant.
Postoperative.
Oestrogens.
Myeloproliferative disease.
Hyperlipidaemia.
Diabetes mellitus.
Cigarette smoking.

Thrombophilia is discussed in the Review articles (Chapter 7).

Final diagnosis

Thrombophilia caused by APCR.

Data interpretation 15

a. Acute leukaemia must be excluded.
Other underlying malignancy.
GI tract bleeding.
Red cell aplasia/haemolysis.
b. Blood film examination for abnormal cells, e.g. lymphoblasts.
Reticulocyte count to exclude haemolysis and aplasia.
Haematinic assays.
Viral serology, especially parvovirus B19.
Consider bone marrow aspirate.

This child had parvovirus B19-induced red cell aplasia. His RCC and reticulocyte counts were low. The blood film showed a mature neutrophilia with no evidence of acute leukaemia. Viral serology confirmed recent parvovirus B19 infection. A bone marrow was not performed but would have shown gross reduction in erythroid elements with normal myeloid and megakaryocytic cell numbers and development. Haematinic assays were normal.

> Parvovirus B19, a DNA virus, causes the childhood exanthem termed fifth disease. The virus invades and destroys developing erythroid cells causing a temporary erythroid aplasia. The aplastic episode generally follows a febrile illness. The disorder may affect children or adults. Recovery is generally rapid with a rebound reticulocytosis.

Final diagnosis

Acute red cell aplasia induced by parvovirus B19 infection.

Data interpretation 16

a. Post-transfusion purpura (PTP).
Consider ITP or drug-induced thrombocytopenia.
b. Obtain preoperative platelet count.
Type patient's platelets for HPA-1a.
Obtain drug history from patient.
c. In view of the severity of the thrombocytopenia admit the patient to hospital until the platelet count is $>10 \times 10^9/l$. Perform a full physical examination including fundoscopy to exclude fundal haemorrhage.
Commence corticosteroids or IVIg.

> PTP is a rare but well-recognized complication of blood transfusion; peak incidence is 5–10 days following blood transfusion. The condition generally affects multiparous women who are negative for the platelet antigen HPA-1a. Sensitization to HPA-1a occurs during previous pregnancies or blood transfusions. Repeat transfusion with HPA-1a positive blood products boosts the alloantibody directed against HPA-1a in the donor blood, which destroys donor platelets and the patient's own platelets at the same time. The mechanism is unclear but it is believed that the patient's own platelets are 'innocent bystanders' and are damaged by immune complexes.
>
> The platelet count usually recovers spontaneously between 3 and 5 weeks. In cases where bleeding or bruising is extensive, steroids (prednisolone 1 mg/kg per day) or IVIg should be started. HPA-1a-negative platelets have been used but without much success and, to date, IVIg appears to be the most effective treatment available.

Final diagnosis

Post-transfusion purpura.

Data interpretation 17

a. CXR.

   Lung function tests.

   Cardiac and abdominal ultrasound.

   Hb electrophoresis.

   Measurement of red cell and plasma volumes.

   Bone marrow aspirate and trephine biopsy.

b. This patient has erythrocytosis and polycythaemia, accounting for his plethoric appearance. Investigation of polycythaemia is often carried out in patients who are middle-aged or older and in whom lung pathology, obesity and primary polycythaemia are commoner than in this patient's age group. In a patient of this age, significant lung pathology through, for example, cigarette smoking is much less likely. A CXR should detect gross lung pathology and some cardiac abnormalities. Lung function tests, although routine, may not add much to the investigative findings in this patient. A cardiac echo would provide evidence of cardiac abnormalities and blood volume studies will confirm true polycythaemia by allowing the measurement of red cell and plasma volumes. In true polycythaemia there will be an elevated red cell mass (as opposed to reduced plasma volume). A bone marrow may demonstrate features suggestive of myeloproliferative disease.

Hb electrophoresis is required to prove that an Hb abnormality is the cause of the polycythaemia. Amino acid changes often lead to alterations in overall charge of the Hb molecule and an abnormal band will be detected on electrophoresis.

This patient had a high-affinity Hb. Such an Hb has a greater affinity for oxygen than normal and shifts the oxygen dissociation curve to the left with compensatory increase in the red cell mass.

> There are 50 or so high-affinity Hbs described to date affecting either the α or β chain of Hb. Examples include Hb Chesapeake, Heathrow, San Diego and many others.
>
> Inheritance is autosomal dominant and those affected are heterozygotes with mild erythrocytosis, which is well tolerated. The homozygous state is probably incompatible with life.
>
> It does not require treatment, although very high PCV levels may occasionally require venesection/phlebotomy.

Final diagnosis

High-affinity Hb resulting in polycythaemia.

Data interpretation 18

a. Hereditary spherocytosis.
b. Aplastic crises.
   Haemolytic crises.
   Gallstones.
c. Hereditary spherocytosis affects 1 : 5000 people and is inherited as an autosomal dominant with variable penetrance in most cases, although autosomal recessive forms have been described. In a quarter of cases there is no family history and these must arise as spontaneous mutations.

   The molecular pathology is complex and highly heterogeneous, but the principal defect is in the spectrin molecule which forms part of the red cell cytoskeleton. In addition, ankyrin, band 3 and protein 4.2 abnormalities play a role. Due to the red cell membrane defect there is increased destruction of red cells (i.e. haemolysis) and formation of spherocytic red cells. Affected red cells are more permeable to Na^+, leading to activation of the Na^+-K^+-ATPase pump and increased K^+ loss.

Presentation can be as mild anaemia in neonates with splenic enlargement and jaundice. Frequently it does not present until adult life, being identified fortuitously on FBC examination for other reasons or presenting as a haemolytic anaemia.

Aplastic crises may be triggered by parvovirus infection. Megaloblastic changes are usually due to folate deficiency consequent upon increased red cell turnover. During infective episodes the haemolysis may increase but it is rarely severe.

Laboratory findings include anaemia, rise in MCHC (50% patients), spherocytic red cells on the film, increased LDH and bilirubin with decreased or absent haptoglobins.

In the osmotic fragility test red cells of the patient and a normal control are tested immediately after drawing the blood and again after 24 h incubation at 37°C (see Fig. 5.1). The osmotic fragility of hereditary spherocytosis red cells is increased when tested immediately and this fragility is exaggerated after 24 h incubation.

Therapy consists of folic acid supplementation, red cell transfusion if required in severe crises, and splenectomy (which corrects anaemia but not the underlying defect; red cell survival is increased in 80% of patients) for more seriously affected individuals.

Final diagnosis

Hereditary spherocytosis.

Data interpretation 19

a. Sepsis.
   DIC secondary to bacterial pathogens.
   CMV infection.
   Toxoplasmosis.
   Rubella.
   Herpes simplex.
   Pre-eclampsia.
   Intrauterine death of a twin.
   Placental abruption.
   Brain injuries.
   Severe hypoxia.
   Shock from any cause.
   Maternal ITP.
   Neonatal alloimmune thrombocytopenia.
b. Observe baby, await normalization of platelet count over the following days or weeks. If bleeding is a problem, consider platelet transfusion (maternal platelets or other HPA-1a-negative platelets) or IVIg.

This baby appears to be well and has normal blood parameters, apart from a reduced platelet count at $2 \times 10^9/l$. Serious infections, hypoxia and shock seem unlikely but a thorough physical examination of the baby should be performed. DIC seems very unlikely, especially since clotting tests are normal and fibrinogen level is normal. Serological tests should be arranged for the viral agents listed and blood cultures taken.

The mother's FBC in the period before delivery should reveal a low platelet count if the mother has ITP; this could affect the baby's platelet count through IgG that crosses the placenta.

> Neonatal alloimmune thrombocytopenia was the cause in this case in a mechanism similar to PTP. The destruction of the baby's platelets is due to an antibody produced by the mother against HPA-1a, one of the platelet antigens. The mother's platelets lack this antigen, which is present on the father's – and hence baby's – platelets.
>
> After sensitization to HPA-1a (e.g. through transfusion or pregnancy) and production of an anamnestic antibody response, the mother produces IgG against HPA-1a which crosses the placenta and causes destruction of the baby's platelets. The mother characteristically has a normal platelet count (cf. maternal or gestational ITP). Testing of the mother's platelets by a regional transfusion centre will confirm that they are HPA-1a-negative.
>
> The antibody is passively transferred to the fetus and the disorder is self-limited; the maternal antibody is gradually cleared from the baby's circulation and the platelet count subsequently rises.

Treatment is only required if the baby is actively bleeding and may consist of transfusion of HPA-1a-negative platelets. Often, washed maternal platelets are given (after all, they are HPA-1a-negative). IVIg may also be used.

The antigen HPA-1a is carried on the platelets of 98% of the population. The remaining few per cent of the population who become pregnant will usually have partners who are HPA-1a-positive as in this case. First-born babies are affected in 50% of cases.

Final diagnosis

Neonatal alloimmune thrombocytopenia.

Data interpretation 20

a. This child has leukopenia and neutropenia. The other FBC indices are normal.
b. Possibilities include:
Drug-induced neutropenia.
Marrow infiltration.
Autoimmune neutropenia.
Congenital neutropenia syndromes:
Kostmann's syndrome.
Transcobalamin II deficiency.
Reticular dysgenesis.
Glycogen storage disease type Ib.
Schwachman-Diamond syndrome.
Chédiak-Higashi syndrome.

This child had Kostmann's syndrome which is inherited in an autosomal recessive manner and gives rise to recurrent infections such as otitis media, enteritis and peritonitis within the first month of life.

The neutrophil count is often very low, as in this case. The bone marrow reveals early myeloid precursors but few intermediate or late neutrophils. There are no karyotypic abnormalities associated with Kostmann's syndrome.

The management is primarily aimed at prevention of infection with antibiotic prophylaxis. G-CSF has been shown to be of benefit in some cases. Cure is possible in patients who undergo allogeneic BMT.

Final diagnosis

Congenital neutropenia (Kostmann's syndrome).

Data interpretation 21

a. Examination of the blood film; this showed polychromasia and large numbers of spherocytes.

   A reticulocyte count. The reticulocytes were significantly elevated at 24%.

   Urinalysis. This showed increased urobilinogen and an absence of biliuria.

   Antiglobulin test. This was negative, ruling out an autoimmune haemolysis.

   A family history should also be obtained. In this case there was no known family history of haematological disorders.

   Viral titres and glandular fever screen should also be checked. Glandular fever screening test was positive and viral screening subsequently confirmed EBV infection.

b. Haemolytic anaemia.

   Causes may be congenital, autoimmune or drug related.

The diagnosis in this case was hereditary spherocytosis; there had been an exacerbation of haemolysis precipitated by infectious mononucleosis. Hereditary spherocytosis may be mild and asymptomatic well into adult life. Exacerbation can be precipitated by viral infection and this viral infection led to the diagnosis of hereditary spherocytosis. Follow-up studies showed increased red cell fragility present in the patient, her sister and her mother, who had no previous medical history.

> Warm antibody autoimmune haemolysis can present a similar clinical picture but is unusual following a viral infection. Infectious mononucleosis may be followed by a transient cold antibody autoimmune haemolysis where cold agglutination would be a feature in the film and the antiglobulin test would be positive with complement coating on the red cells. Drug-related haemolysis is possible given that she had been exposed to mefenamic acid. Mefenamic acid is occasionally reported as causing autoimmune haemolysis but usually in large doses as the result of an idiosyncratic immune complex reaction.
>
> Management of acute haemolysis in hereditary spherocytosis is essentially supportive. Supplementary folic acid to compensate for the increased demands is usually given, including long-term administration. If patients become symptomatically anaemic, supportive transfusion may be needed. Current practice would avoid splenectomy except for patients who are chronically debilitated by recurrent haemolysis or with massive splenomegaly.

Final diagnosis

Hereditary spherocytosis haemolytic crisis, exacerbated by infectious mononucleosis.

Data interpretation 22

a. The clinical features and abnormal clotting tests appear to indicate an acquired disorder of haemostasis. The combination of prolongation in the PT and APTT most commonly results from the effect of oral anticoagulants or severe liver disease. Heparin effect or a dysfibrinogenaemia could also produce such abnormalities.

b. Confirmation of the abnormalities with a repeat sample to rule out any technical problems in sampling would be reasonable. The pattern of abnormalities was confirmed. Correction (mixing) experiments should be requested. Addition of 50% normal plasma to the patient's plasma sample produced correction of the clotting abnormalities. This phenomenon effectively rules out the presence of an inhibitor. Thrombin clotting time could also be carried out; this was normal, indicating a normal effective fibrinogen level and lack of a heparin effect.

Clinical assessment and history gave no indication that underlying liver disease or alcohol abuse were likely contributory factors.

c. Having confirmed clotting factor deficiencies, replacement with fresh frozen plasma was undertaken. After 2 units of fresh frozen plasma there was partial correction of the clotting abnormalities and the bleeding stabilized. Some 24 h after 2 units of fresh frozen plasma, there was still prolongation of the PT and APTT. There was no bleeding and the test was repeated 24 h later, when the results were almost fully back to normal.

The diagnosis in this case was cryptic warfarin ingestion. The patient in question was a nurse and had a history of recent psychiatric problems. Once liver disease has been excluded and the possibility of heparin effect has been eliminated, there is virtually no other known explanation for prolongation of both PT and APTT.

Final diagnosis

Cryptic warfarin ingestion.

Data interpretation 23

a. Generalized malabsorption states:
   Coeliac disease.
   Crohn's disease.
   Whipple's disease.
   Pancreatic insufficiency.
   Protein-losing enteropathy.
   Tropical sprue.
b. Upper GI tract endoscopy and duodenal biopsies.
c. Small-bowel lymphoma/carcinoma (especially of the oesophagus).
   Intestinal ulcers and strictures.
   Dermatitis herpetiformis.

This patient was mildly anaemic with macrocytosis. The film features suggested vitamin B_{12} and/or folate deficiency and these were confirmed by the haematinic assays. The fact that B_{12}, folate and ferritin were reduced suggests an underlying malabsorption state. This was made more likely given the history of weight loss, frequent passage of stools and the finding of finger clubbing. The biochemistry profile also showed hypocalcaemia, again in keeping with malabsorption. The diagnosis was coeliac disease.

Coeliac disease is typically associated with deficiencies of iron and folate but B_{12} deficiency is also described. The disorder is not well understood in terms of aetiology and pathogenesis but gluten sensitivity has been shown to cause damage to intestinal epithelium in these patients. Genetic factors probably play a role, with increased incidence of the disease in first-degree relatives. Some 70–80% of patients are HLA-B8 and DW3-positive (cf. 20% of the general population).

The clinical features include diarrhoea, weight loss and abdominal bloating. The diagnosis requires small-bowel biopsy. This will show subtotal villous atrophy, crypt hypertrophy and inflammatory cell infiltrate. IgG and IgA antigliadin antibodies are elevated in 90% of patients.

Treatment is straightforward and entails avoidance of gluten-containing foods, which means eliminating wheat, rye, oats and barley from the diet. The only flour allowed is rice and corn flour.

Final diagnosis

Combined vitamin B_{12}, folate and iron deficiencies secondary to coeliac disease.

Data interpretation 24

a. The patient had prolongation of the APTT with a normal PT. On the addition of normal plasma there is shortening but not complete correction of the APTT, suggesting that there is an inhibitor in the patient's plasma.
b. Inhibitor assay.

Unlike haemophilia A, the inhibitors affect both males and females. Autoantibodies against clotting factors are well described. Antibodies against FVIII are commonest; these are predominantly IgG and are directed primarily against the FVIII procoagulant activity. Antibodies against FVIII are seen also in haemophilia A (15–25% of young patients). In non-haemophilic adults autoantibodies against FVIII are seen in pregnancy and the postpartum period, autoimmune disease (e.g. rheumatoid, SLE, Crohn's, myasthenia gravis), solid tumours and drug reactions.

Clinical presentation of patients with acquired inhibitors to FVIII tends to be fairly dramatic, with sudden onset of bruising, bleeding into joints, severe epistaxes and GI bleeding. Investigations show an elevation of the APTT which does not correct with the addition of normal plasma. Further investigation needs to be carried out to confirm the presence of an inhibitor.

> If the investigations confirm the presence of an FVIII inhibitor then immunosuppression may be of value, especially in the presence of bleeding. Drugs used include oral prednisolone with or without cyclophosphamide. In severe bleeds porcine FVIII (to which the autoantibody should not react) may be given. Other treatment modalities include plasmapheresis, desmopressin (DDAVP), activated FIX complex, IVIg and recombinant factor VIIa.

Final diagnosis

Autoimmune FVIII inhibitor associated with rheumatoid disease.

Data interpretation 25

a. This woman had a reduced Hb and low MCV. The film showed target and pencil cells suggestive of possible underlying iron deficiency. The MCV was very low and, in fact, much too low for the degree of anaemia simply to be due to iron deficiency alone. This would suggest an underlying haemoglobin disorder such as thalassaemia, e.g. β-thalassaemia trait.

b. Hb electrophoresis would be useful to confirm the presence of haemoglobinopathy. It would also be useful to screen her partner and children for the presence of an abnormal Hb.

c. This woman could have been iron-deficient with an underlying haemoglobinopathy; however serum ferritin estimation proved normal.

She needs no treatment for underlying β-thalassaemia trait but her partner needs to be screened. If he carries the β-thalassaemia mutation then their children have a 25% chance of having thalassaemia major, a debilitating disease requiring regular blood transfusion and associated with iron overload, etc.

> In fact, Hb electrophoresis was performed and this woman was found to have an elevated HbA$_2$ of 5.5% (normal <2%), indicative of β-thalassaemia trait. Her HbF was normal (<1%). The serum ferritin was not indicative of iron deficiency and the mild anaemia was judged to be in keeping with the underlying β-thalassaemia trait. Her excessive tiredness was attributed to stress/anxiety with no major organic cause likely.

The mildest form of β-thalassaemia is β-thalassaemia trait, in which there is one normal β-globin gene and one thalassaemic β-globin gene. The mutated β-globin gene may produce reduced β chains (β$^+$-thalassaemia) or no β-globin (β^o-thalassaemia). In general, β-thalassaemia trait is a mild disorder with few symptoms. Most patients are not anaemic (or are only mildly anaemic) and demonstrate no abnormal clinical signs. The disorder is common in Italy, Greece, Cyprus, India, Thailand and south-east Asia.

Despite the relatively normal Hb, the MCV is usually very low and the peripheral blood film may not show any hypochromic changes. Target cells may be conspicuous on the blood film. Basophilic red cell stippling may be seen. Reticulocytes are often increased.

The thalassaemias are inherited abnormalities of globin synthesis. In α-thalassaemia there is impaired α chain production and in β-thalassaemia there is impairment of β-globin synthesis. The hallmark of thalassaemia is impaired production of one globin with excess of other globin chains. This results in precipitation of the excess globin and reduced red cell survival (haemolysis). In β-thalassaemia point mutations are the predominant underlying cause of reduced β-globin production (cf. α-thalassaemia where a gene deletion is more common). Reduced β-globin production leads to a reduction in HbA ($\alpha_2\beta_2$) with a rise in HbA$_2$ ($\alpha_2\delta_2$) and

HbF ($\alpha_2\gamma_2$), since they contain other β-like chains. The overall result is a microcytic anaemia. Due to the α:β globin chain imbalance the excess α chains precipitate leading to inhibition of normal cellular processes, resulting in phagocytosis and destruction of developing red cells within the bone marrow (ineffective erythropoiesis). The extent of anaemia in β-thalassaemia depends on the degree of suppression of β-chain production.

Hb electrophoresis allows HbA$_2$ to be estimated. In β-thalassaemia the HbA$_2$ is always elevated. In around 30% of patients, HbF is also increased. Diagnosis of the trait in pregnancy is more difficult since the indices are less characteristic (e.g. MCV rises in pregnancy). Various formulae have been developed to attempt to differentiate thalassaemia trait from iron deficiency, e.g. MCV ÷ RCC <13 suggests β-thalassaemia trait whilst a figure of >13.3 suggests iron-deficiency anaemia; none has proved reliable in clinical practice.

Final diagnosis

β-thalassaemia trait.

Data interpretation 26

a. Peripheral blood cell surface markers.
   Bone marrow aspirate and trephine biopsy.
   Diagnostic and therapeutic splenectomy.
b. Prolymphocytic leukaemia. In this case the diagnosis was confirmed by splenectomy and cell surface markers.

Prolymphocytic leukaemia, a low-grade B cell neoplasm, has an incidence about 10% that of CLL.

Fifty per cent of patients with prolymphocytic leukaemia present over the age of 70 years. Massive splenomegaly with minimal palpable lymphadenopathy is often found. More than 75% of patients have blood lymphocyte counts > 100 × 10^9/l. The prolymphocytic leukaemic cells have high levels of surface immunoglobulin; 50% are CD5$^+$ and also CD20$^+$ and CD22$^+$. One-third of patients have a monoclonal band on serum protein electrophoresis.

A minority of cases (20%) are T cell in origin: 75% are CD4$^+$, 20% are CD8$^+$ and 15% are CD4$^+$ CD8$^+$.

Abnormalities of chromosome 14q$^+$ occur in 60% of cases.

The disease is typically resistant to chlorambucil. Combination chemotherapy in the form of CHOP may produce a response (complete or partial) in 50% of patients but the responses are short-lived. The purine analogues (e.g. fludarabine) may be a useful therapeutic alternative.

Splenectomy is performed in some cases and may ameliorate the symptoms but this effect is usually transient. Splenic irradiation may be used in patients who are poor candidates for chemotherapy and/or splenectomy.

The median survival for B prolymphocytic leukaemia is 3 years (cf. CLL at 8 years); in T prolymphocytic leukaemia the median survival is even poorer, at 6–7 months.

Final diagnosis

B cell prolymphocytic leukaemia.

Data interpretation 27

a. Stasis in the peripheral (cooler) circulation secondary to red cell agglutination.

b. The blood count shows spurious indices, since the blood cell counter has assessed clumps of red cells rather than single red cells. In the laboratory, spontaneous red cell agglutination is frequently observed both macroscopically and on the peripheral blood film. Red cell agglutinates can often be dispersed by warming of the blood sample prior to making the blood film and performing the automated cell count.

The blood count shows an anaemia with reticulocytosis and lymphocytosis. This pattern is suggestive of an autoimmune haemolytic anaemia due to a cold-type antibody. The lymphocytosis raises the possibility of an underlying viral illness or lymphoproliferative disorder.

c. Direct antiglobulin test.

Detection of cold agglutinins and determination of titre and specificity.

Full infection screen (to include *Mycoplasma pneumoniae* and EBV) and Monospot test for infectious mononucleosis.

Investigations to look for an underlying lymphoma (serum protein electrophoresis; bone marrow examination; whole-body imaging, etc.).

d. The mainstay of management is to keep the patient warm (especially the extremities). Folic acid should be given as for any chronic haemolytic state. Blood transfusion may be indicated during acute haemolytic exacerbations, but should be administrated through a blood warmer. Glucocorticoids and splenectomy are not generally helpful. However, alkylating agents (chlorambucil, cyclophosphamide) may help in cases of active haemolysis by decreasing the antibody production. In severely ill patients, plasmapheresis may provide temporary relief by removing antibody from the circulation.

The post-infectious syndromes are self-limiting but if cold agglutinin-mediated autoimmune haemolytic anaemia is the result of an underlying lymphoma, then the lymphoma will need treatment in its own right.

Cold agglutinins are usually complement-fixing IgM autoantibodies which are lytic *in vitro* and may cause severe intravascular haemolysis *in vivo*. The specificity of cold agglutinins is usually directed against I/i antigens on the red cells and in cold agglutinin-mediated haemolysis, the direct antiglobulin test is positive with anticomplement reagents only (the IgM readily dissociates from the red cells *in vitro*).

Cold agglutinin-mediated haemolysis accounts for 10–20% of all cases of autoimmune haemolytic anaemia. It may be primary – idiopathic cold haemagglutinin disease – which is a syndrome mainly of the elderly with a monoclonal IgM cold agglutinin, classically with anti-I specificity. It may be considered as a special form of monoclonal gammopathy, and runs a chronic and usually benign course. Cold agglutinin-mediated haemolysis can be secondary to underlying lymphoproliferative disorders (monoclonal IgM with either anti-I or anti-i specificity) or to infections such as *Mycoplasma pneumoniae* (polyclonal IgM with anti-I specificity) and infectious mononucleosis (polyclonal IgM with anti-i specificity).

The patient presented here had cold agglutinin-mediated haemolysis associated with an underlying NHL of low-grade subtype. Both conditions responded well to antilymphoma therapy.

Final diagnosis

Cold haemagglutinin-mediated haemolysis secondary to lymphoproliferative disorder.

Data interpretation 28

a. PNH.
b. Serum bilirubin and LDH.
   Ham's acid lysis test.
   Serum haptoglobins.
   Urinary haemosiderin.
   Serum ferritin.
c. Red cell complement-mediated lysis.

The combination of venous thrombosis and haemolysis with pancytopenia is very suggestive of PNH. PNH is an intrinsic red cell disorder that is clonal and acquired. The clone arises in a marrow that has undergone previous damage and may follow aplastic anaemia or other marrow injury. Chromosomal analysis shows a normal karyotype in most cases. Classical PNH is characterized by increased sensitivity of the red cells to complement-mediated lysis (hence Ham's acid lysis test is positive). The dark urine, a hallmark of this disorder, may be passed at any time of day but typically follows sleep. This was previously believed to be due to a lowering of the blood pH, but this has been shown not to be the case.

Patients with PNH demonstrate features of chronic haemolysis with associated weakness, dyspnoea, pallor and splenomegaly in some cases. Iron deficiency is common (note the low MCV in this patient) but macrocytosis is a common finding due to the accompanying reticulocytosis. Bleeding may be present and severe if thrombocytopenia is severe. Thrombosis is common but the exact mechanism underlying this is unclear. Both arterial and venous thrombosis have been reported. Renal manifestations may take the form of abnormal tubular function and diminished creatinine clearance.

Laboratory features include anaemia, mild/moderate reticulocytosis and macrocytosis. The WBC is generally low. The platelets may be low but are normal in 20% of patients. The marrow shows erythroid hyperplasia. Hb casts may be present in the urine. Haemosiderinuria is one of the most constant features of the disease and is of great diagnostic importance.

The underlying defect is in the X-linked phosphatidyl inositol glycan class A (PIG-A) gene, which participates in an early step of GPI anchor synthesis in the red cell. Other proteins are probably involved in the pathogenesis of PNH. The result is that those cell surface proteins that are normally attached via this anchor to the membrane are deficient in PNH-affected cells. It appears that reduced expression of one such protein, CD59, is the major reason for the sensitivity of red cells to complement. Treatment is essentially supportive, with blood transfusions, antibiotics and anticoagulants. Some patients may benefit from BMT. Development of AML may be seen in a minority of patients with PNH.

Final diagnosis

PNH.

Data interpretation 29

a. Bleeding time.
   ESR or plasma viscosity.
   MSU.
   Skin biopsy.
   Autoimmune profile.
b. This patient seems to have a purpuric rash, with colicky abdominal pain, melaena and fever following one episode of upper respiratory infection. His clotting screen was normal and he had a normal bleeding time. Because of the abnormal urea and creatinine, an MSU was requested and it revealed microscopic haematuria, proteinuria and red cell casts. His ESR was mildly elevated. The most likely diagnosis in this age group is Henoch–Schönlein or allergic purpura. The differential diagnosis includes SLE, polyarteritis and essential cryoglobulinaemia.

c. In most patients the disease remits spontaneously. Glucocorticoids (prednisolone 1 mg/kg per day) are effective in controlling the arthralgia and the abdominal pain during the acute illness. In chronic renal disease immunosuppressive therapy with azathioprine has been reported to be of value. Plasma exchange has also been tried in resistant cases.

Allergic purpura is usually seen in children and young adults (mean age 6–7 years) following infection, drugs, certain foods, bites or immunizations. Henoch–Schönlein purpura is a systemic disease with a tendency to resolve and recur several times over a period of weeks or months. The typical purpura is seen in almost all patients. GI involvement is very frequent in children and it may be complicated by intussusception of the intestine. The renal involvement is characterized by a mild glomerulonephritis leading to haematuria with red cell casts. The disorder is associated with perivascular inflammatory lesions with serosanginous leakage into skin, submucosal and serosal areas. The lesions produced are palpable, symmetrical and affect the distal extremities. Renal biopsy shows mild diffuse mesangial prominence; some cases demonstrate focal segmental proliferative glomerulonephritis. When studied by immunofluorescence techniques there are mesangial deposits that are reactive for IgA, C3 and C5 complement components. Arthritis tends to be non-deforming. Laboratory findings are non-specific. Elevated IgA is frequently reported. Serum complement levels are normal. Platelet counts are normal.

The course is variable. The 15-year survival in children is 90%. Some 15% have persistent disease and 8% demonstrate renal impairment.

Final diagnosis

Henoch-Schönlein purpura.

Data interpretation 30

a. Differential diagnosis is that of a macrocytic anaemia in a 67-year-old. Given the history of anaemia some 6 years ago treated with vitamin B_{12} it may be simply that she had developed recurrent vitamin B_{12} deficiency because of failure to continue with replacement therapy. In the absence of further detail about her previous anaemia, this would remain a genuine possibility; the total WBC and platelet count are less in favour of a presentation of vitamin B_{12} deficiency since these usually start to reduce as the anaemia becomes more severe. Folic acid deficiency requires to be considered as the haematological indices are indistinguishable from those of vitamin B_{12} deficiency.

Macrocytosis with a history of previous anaemia and Dupuytren's contracture should also raise the suspicion of a high alcohol intake. Myelodysplasia can present as a macrocytic anaemia and requires to be excluded; the normal white cell and platelet counts are not totally in favour of this diagnosis, especially the apparent lack of dysplastic white cell changes. Hypothyroidism should also be considered in an elderly person with macrocytic anaemia and is easily checked. The clinical features are less suggestive of this, especially the presence of physiological tendon jerks. Liver disease would also be a possibility, although target cells would be expected on the blood film and other clinical stigmata are not clearly present.

b. Further investigations were done. Vitamin B_{12}, folate and ferritin were carried out. Vitamin B_{12} was normal at 187 ng/l, red cell folate was reduced at 119 μg/l (normal 150–700 μg/l), serum folate was reduced at 0.9 μg/l (normal 2.0–11.0 μg/l). Ferritin was normal at 119 μg/l. Urea and electrolytes were normal. LFTs demonstrated a bilirubin of 5 μmol/l, alkaline phosphatase 255 i.u./l, albumin 33 g/l and a total protein of 72 g/l. LDH was requested and was elevated at 548 i.u./l and gamma glutamyl transferase was 42 i.u./l (normal 10–46 i.u./l). Thyroid function was normal; free T_4 was 11.6 pmol/l. Bone marrow aspirate was carried out and showed hyperplasia of all elements with predominant erythroid hyperplasia and definite megaloblastic change. Iron stores were abundant.

The most important investigation was a review of her diet and social history and obtaining information from her daughter. She had given a vague dietary history and had suggested that her overall nutrition was poor. She admitted to drinking two or three glasses of sherry per day. Her daughter emphasized that her diet was grossly deficient in virtually all nutritional categories and that her consumption of sherry was somewhat higher – she estimated an average consumption of a bottle of sherry per day. This had been previously identified with the anaemia 6 years ago. No evidence of vitamin B_{12} deficiency or pernicious anaemia had been identified; she had given up alcohol for some 2–3 years but had resumed her present pattern thereafter.

Haematological features are therefore those of alcohol excess with associated dietary folate deficiency. Alcohol may produce a range of haematological changes. Most common is a macrocytosis in the absence of anaemia due to a direct effect on bone marrow and red cells. Poor nutrition resulting in folate deficiency, as in this case, can occur. Alcohol excess can produce a megaloblastic-like state and quite severe degrees of anaemia in extremely heavy drinkers.

A rare haemolytic anaemia accompanied by hyperlipidaemia (Zieve's syndrome) can occur. It usually occurs in chronic alcoholics and follows binge drinking. Alcohol will also produce coagulation abnormalities as a result of liver disease. Leukopenia and thrombocytopenia may also be produced by alcohol excess.

Final diagnosis

Folate deficiency and alcohol abuse.

Data interpretation 31

a. Haemolytic anaemia secondary to presence of a heart valve prosthesis, i.e. traumatic cardiac haemolytic anaemia.
b. DCT (DAT).
   Estimation of serum LDH, serum haptoglobins and urine for haemosiderin.
   Clotting screen, including fibrinogen and fibrin degradation products.
   Serum ferritin.
   Echocardiogram to assess function of the prosthetic valve and overall myocardial efficiency.
c. Folic acid and iron supplements for mild compensated intravascular haemolysis with urinary iron loss. In severe haemolysis blood transfusion may be required and surgical replacement of the prosthesis should be considered. If surgery is contraindicated, propranolol may help to decrease shear forces between the prosthesis and red blood cells. rHuEPO may have a role in reducing transfusion requirements.

Traumatic cardiac haemolytic anaemia due to valve prostheses has become very uncommon as non-thrombogenic valves have superseded the older plastic or metal mechanical valves. It is very occasionally seen in severe aortic or subaortic stenosis that has not been surgically treated. The haemolysis is usually mild and well compensated and the DCT test is negative. Red cell destruction is intravascular and results in haemoglobinaemia, haemoglobinuria and haemosiderinuria. Urinary iron loss may lead to a state of iron deficiency.

In situations where there is red cell fragmentation on the blood film, it is important to exclude DIC and clotting studies are essential. In this case, the normal platelet count makes DIC very unlikely. However, it is worth remembering that the platelet count may be reduced in cases such as this due to formation of platelet thrombi on abnormal valve surfaces.

The cardiac status must be assessed, as traumatic cardiac haemolytic anaemia often reflects a leaking or otherwise faulty prosthesis and there may be evidence of cardiac failure which may require specific therapy.

Final diagnosis

Haemolytic anaemia secondary to heart valve prosthesis.

Data interpretation 32

a. LFTs would be of value. These should include γ-glutamyl transferase, alanine aminotransferase and serum bilirubin. Deranged clotting along with abnormalities of these liver enzymes would suggest liver pathology, e.g. secondary to alcohol consumption.

Mixing studies or correction tests would be useful in this man. These involve mixing the patient's plasma with normal plasma in a 50 : 50 ratio. Normal plasma will provide all the required clotting factors necessary for coagulation *in vitro*. Therefore, if the clotting tests become normal after adding normal plasma then the abnormal results are due to deficiency of a clotting factor. If no correction (or partial correction only) occurs then it is possible that there is an inhibitor in the patient's plasma, e.g. lupus anticoagulant.

b. Hepatic dysfunction with coagulopathy secondary to alcohol consumption. A viral aetiology should be considered, especially in a patient who has travelled abroad as was the case here, e.g. viral hepatitis or haemorrhagic fever (unlikely since this patient was actually quite well).

Final diagnosis

Liver dysfunction secondary to alcohol abuse.

Data interpretation 33

a. ALL. The morphological details suggest that this is ALL L1 in the FAB classification and the marker studies show that this is of the pre-BALL variety (cALLA$^+$ HLA class II$^+$ surface Ig$^-$). The cells expressing T cell antigens represent the normal T cells and demonstrate that lymphocytes make up approximately 30% of the blood mononuclear cells.

b. Bone marrow aspirate for morphology, cytochemical stains, cell marker analysis, and cytogenetic assessment.
Bone marrow trephine biopsy.
Lumbar puncture and cytospin preparation to exclude CNS involvement by leukaemic blasts.

c. Age (most favourable age is between 2 and 12 years).
WBC at presentation ($<50 \times 10^9/l$ more favourable).
Sex (female sex favourable).
Presence of CNS disease (adverse feature).
Cytogenetic status (normal cytogenetics and hyperdiploidy indicate good prognosis; the Philadelphia translocation and 11q23 abnormalities indicate poor prognosis).

ALL has its greatest incidence under 10 years of age and bone pain is a very common presenting feature, particularly in children. The diagnosis may be obvious from the peripheral blood features (as in this case), but a bone marrow aspirate is always necessary to confirm the diagnosis and allow a precise classification.

ALL blast cells are usually PAS$^+$ and TdT$^+$ while myeloperoxidase and non-specific stains are usually negative. Bone marrow trephine is an important investigation, especially in those instances where the aspirate may not be representative of the extent of the disease (for example in hypercellular, dense hypercellular or fibrotic cases). A CXR should always be performed since a mediastinal mass is present in 50% cases with T cell ALL.

The overall prognosis for childhood ALL is now very good, with expectation of cure in more than 60% of patients. However, these results are only achieved with complex treatment protocols, involving intensive chemotherapy for remission induction and consolidation, prophylactic or therapeutic treatment of CNS with chemo-radiotherapy and a prolonged period of maintenance therapy with further cytotoxic drugs.

The Philadelphia chromosome is associated with ~95% of cases of CML, 1–2% of cases of childhood ALL and 15–20% of adult ALL. As mentioned above, the presence of the Philadelphia chromosome in ALL is an adverse prognostic factor.

Final diagnosis

ALL; cALL subtype.

Data interpretation 34

a. Mixing tests (50 : 50 mix of normal plasma with patient's plasma) with repeat APTT.
   Lupus anticoagulant (e.g. DRVVT).
   Anticardiolipin assay.
   Autoimmune profile.
b. Consider lifelong warfarin.

This young woman has two documented thrombotic events and possibly a third. The FBC is normal but clotting tests are clearly abnormal. The PT is normal but APTT is significantly prolonged, suggesting an abnormality of the intrinsic pathway. This can occur due to either deficiency of a coagulation factor or the presence of an inhibitor.

If the prolongation is due to deficiency, then mixing the patient's plasma with normal plasma should correct the APTT to normal. If, however, the prolongation is due to an inhibitor then on mixing patient with normal plasma there will still be a long APTT. She was diagnosed as having the lupus anticoagulant.

Lupus anticoagulant prolongs the APTT but predisposes to thrombosis rather than bleeding and increases the risk of arterial and venous thromboembolism.

> The laboratory confirmation of lupus anticoagulant is the DTT, which is based on the PT. Characteristically divergent lines are produced when comparing control with patient plasma (Fig. 6.2). In addition, some patients may have anti-cardiolipin antibodies (IgG or IgA or both) and the presence of these in patients with SLE correlates more strongly with thrombosis and fetal loss than clotting assays for lupus anticoagulant alone.
>
> Lupus anticoagulant is not associated purely with SLE and many patients with lupus anticoagulant have no evidence of SLE. Lupus anticoagulant has been documented in other autoimmune disorders, after ingestion of various drugs, infections, malignancy, and in apparently normal individuals.
>
> Warfarin is effective in preventing further thrombosis and should be considered in this patient.

Final diagnosis

Lupus anticoagulant syndrome.

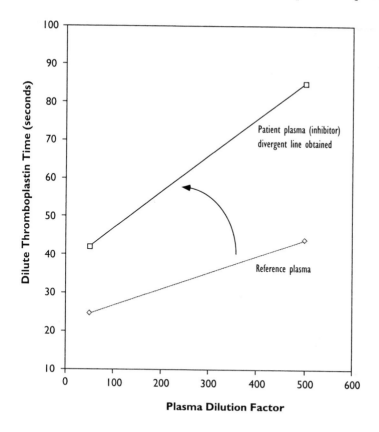

Fig. 6.2   Patient and control (reference) plasmas assayed using DTT: in deficiency the lines are parallel; in presence of lupus inhibitor the lines are divergent

Data interpretation 35

a. Transformation of previous low-grade NHL to large-cell NHL (i.e. from low-to high-grade disease).
b. Ascitic tap.
CT scan of the chest and abdomen.
Serum LDH level.
Bone marrow aspirate and trephine biopsy.

> Follicular lymphoma is the commonest subtype of NHL encountered in clinical practice. Patients are generally middle-aged with painless and slowly progressive lymphadenopathy. 'B' symptoms (e.g. weight loss and night sweats) may be present but if severe or of sudden onset should raise suspicions of transformation of previous low-grade disease to a high-grade NHL, as in this case. Other features suggestive of transformation include rapid enlargement of lymph nodes.

Treatment is essentially palliative and the disease has a median survival of 7 years. The disorder is incurable and most patients die from their disease. Treatment is indicated for systemic symptoms, obstructive lymphadenopathy, marrow failure, etc. and may consist of local radiotherapy for localized disease or systemic chemotherapy for widespread disease. Combination chemotherapy (e.g. CHOP) may result in a faster response but survival is unchanged.

The hallmark of follicular NHL is the cytogenetic abnormality t(14;18) involving the immunoglobulin gene locus and bcl-2 gene. This results in a reduction in apoptosis (programmed cell death) and may be instrumental in the pathology of the disease.

This woman demonstrated features of progression to high-grade NHL. The raised serum calcium is in keeping with this diagnosis. The ascites should also raise suspicions about the possibility of development of a second cancer (e.g. ovarian) following alkylating agent administration. In fact, she only had four previous courses of chemotherapy and therefore this was felt unlikely. Nevertheless, the development of secondary cancers must be considered in patients who have been given prolonged courses of alkylating agents.

Final diagnosis

Transformation of low-grade to high-grade NHL.

Data interpretation 36

a. β-thalassaemia intermedia.
b. This patient appears to have β-thalassaemia of a severity greater than thalassaemia trait but with an age of onset later than β-thalassaemia major. He is able to survive without regular blood transfusion and has grown normally. Although the analysis and quantitation of the haemoglobins suggest homozygous β°-thalassaemia, the clinically milder disorder indicates that he has β-thalassaemia intermedia.

β-thalassaemia intermedia is a clinically heterogeneous disorder and there are a number of genetic factors that may result in this phenotype. Among these are the inheritance of 'mild' forms of β-thalassaemia (β^{+}, where some β chains are produced), the co-inheritance of various forms of α-thalassaemia, and the inheritance of an enhanced propensity for HbF production (including δβ-thalassaemia and hereditary persistence of HbF).

c. In the absence of systemic symptoms or features, it is preferable to avoid embarking on a regular transfusion regimen. These patients can often manage with only occasional transfusions for episodes of symptomatic anaemia. If splenomegaly develops, as in this case, it may compound the anaemia by causing haemodilution and pooling. Splenectomy is then often beneficial and it may render a patient transfusion-independent.

Iron overload, due to increased absorption and blood transfusion, is a feature of β-thalassaemia intermedia and body iron status should be periodically assessed. Gentle venesection may be able to control iron excess but often chelation therapy with desferrioxamine is required.

Final diagnosis

β-Thalassaemia intermedia.

Data interpretation 37

a. Diagnoses to consider include:
   Hodgkin's disease.
   Mediastinal germ cell tumour.
   Large cell NHL.
   Lymphoblastic lymphoma.
b. FBC.
   CT-guided biopsy of the mediastinal mass.
   Serum α-fetoprotein and human chorionic gonadotrophin levels.
   Bone marrow aspirate and trephine biopsy.

This patient had obviously rapidly advancing disease and the differential diagnoses are listed above. The ultimate diagnostic test is the biopsy of the affected tissue, and in this case CT-guided biopsy of the chest wall lesion was performed. This confirmed a diagnosis of large cell NHL.

The disease was treated with systemic combination chemotherapy and localized DXT and the SVC obstruction resolved rapidly. Complete remission was obtained and, following 6 cycles of treatment, the patient remains in complete remission more than 2 years after initial diagnosis.

Final diagnosis

Large cell NHL.

Data interpretation 38

a. Father was A Rh D-positive.
Mother was O Rh D-negative.
Baby was A Rh D-positive.
The DCT on the baby's red cells was positive.

> The maternal serum contained anti-D plus anti-Le[a] (see panel Chapter 5, Fig. 5.2).

b. The diagnosis is Rh D HDN and possible ABO HDN.

> Anti-Le[a], which is a naturally occurring antibody in Le[a]-negative individuals but can also be formed after transfusion or pregnancy, will not contribute to HDN in the neonate.

c. Blood transfused should be group O Rh D-negative. In order to avoid aggravating any possible ABO HDN, the maternal serum should be screened for high-titre anti-A, and if positive, the donor red cells should be resuspended in AB plasma.

Final diagnosis

Rhesus D HDN.

Data interpretation 39

a. There has been a delayed transfusion reaction. The patient and all donor red cells were group O Rhesus D-negative. Two of the three donor units were Jk[a]-positive. The patient had no detectable anti-Jk[a] in her pre-transfusion sample, but has anti-Jk[a] in the post-transfusion sample, which was also DCT-positive.

b. Blood lacking the Jk[a] antigen should be used for further transfusion.

> There has been a delayed haemolytic transfusion reaction due to anti-Jk[a] which was not detected in the pre-transfusion sample. Exposure to Jk[a] antigens in the transfused blood produced a secondary response which was easily detectable in the post-transfusion sample and which also caused the positive DCT and the symptoms.

Final diagnosis

Delayed haemolytic transfusion reaction.

Data interpretation 40

a. She had a microcytic hypochromic anaemia. The MCV is very low, in keeping with a diagnosis of iron-deficiency anaemia, but the Hb is not as low as one might expect for an MCV of 58 fl. Haemoglobinopathies such as β-thalassaemia would lead to indices such as these and, although not common in northern Europeans, β-thalassaemia does occur in these populations. This woman, however, had normal indices 3 years previously. The WBC is elevated, mainly due to neutrophilia in response to the infection. Her platelets were reduced.

b. The FBC should be repeated to ensure that the indices are correct.

Haematinics should be checked (serum ferritin, vitamin B_{12} and folate).

Bone marrow aspirate and trephine biopsy should be carried out since she has unusual indices and there were teardrop red cells noted in the film, perhaps suggestive of infiltration of the marrow or underlying MDS, not uncommon in patients of this age.

> In fact, this woman had myelodysplasia. This resulted in a reduced Hb and platelet count. Her indices were normal previously, which makes an inherited disorder such as thalassaemia extremely unlikely. A bone marrow was performed and this showed dysplastic changes in all three cell lines (red cells, myeloid cells and megakaryocytes). This explains the falling Hb and platelet count. Hb electrophoresis was carried out and this confirmed the presence of HbH ($β_4$ tetramers).
>
> HbH is typical of α thalassaemia whereby a reduction in α-globin production leads to excess β chains that form tetramers ($β_4$). As an acquired abnormality HbH may be found in patients with MDS. The indices are typically microcytic and hypochromic with basophilic stippling (dyserythropoiesis) and target cells. Crystal violet stains the HbH and produces so-called H bodies identical to those found in α-thalassaemia.
>
> The mechanism of HbH is quite different to that found in α-thalassaemia since there is no gene deletion involved in HbH associated with MDS. Instead, α-globin is simply produced at a reduced rate in erythroblasts, leading to $β_4$ formation.

Final diagnosis

Acquired HbH in MDS.

7 Review articles

Evaluation of anaemia and the FBC

Data from an FBC are frequently extensive and confusing. It is important, therefore, to have a simplified, systematic approach to interpret full FBC data. For the clinician the key initial values to note in determining red cell abnormalities are the Hb level and the MCV. The MCV is determined accurately by modern automated blood counters and for practical purposes supercedes the red cell indices, the MCH and the MCHC.

The normal range for adult Hb is 13.0–18.0 g/dl for a male and 11.5–16.0 g/dl for a female. There are some variations in the normal range for MCV depending on blood counter and normal population. The lower limit of MCV is generally 76–80 fl. and the upper limit 96–100 fl. Using the Hb and MCV will provide effective 'triage' of blood count results.

If the MCV is reduced then the likely causes are iron-deficiency anaemia, thalassaemia trait and secondary, chronic disorder anaemias. Further investigation will obviously depend on clinical circumstances. Finding a very low Hb and MCV in a female aged 37 with a history of menorrhagia makes iron deficiency very likely. Finding a Hb marginally reduced with a very low MCV in an otherwise fit 20-year-old raises the possibility of β-thalassaemia. In most circumstances confirmatory testing for iron deficiency is advisable to complement clinical evaluation.

Anaemias in which the MCV is normal are usually not due to haematinic deficiency. Most commonly they are secondary, non-specific associations with underlying systemic disease. Recent or active bleeding will also produce an anaemia in which the MCV can be expected to be normal. Raised MCV in the absence of anaemia is very common in excessive alcohol intake. Cytotoxic drug therapy, particularly antimetabolites and hydroxyurea, may produce elevation of the MCV. Thyroid disease may produce macrocytosis. Liver dysfunction will frequently be associated with a raised MCV. Marked elevation of the MCV can be found in megaloblastic anaemias of B_{12} and folate deficiency. A major group of conditions in which macrocytosis is a feature is MDS. Macrocytosis may be an early presentation of myelodysplasia, especially in the elderly. Other marrow disorders, including aplastic anaemia, may present with a marginal elevation of the MCV. Haemolytic states with a marked reticulocytosis can cause macrocytosis.

The PCV or haematocrit is not typically used in assessment of anaemia in the UK, although the haematocrit assumes increasing importance in the monitoring of polycythaemic states. The MCHC and MCH fall in association with the MCV in iron-deficiency anaemia. In hereditary spherocytosis and other spherocytic haemolytic anaemias the MCHC may be increased.

Assessment of the white cell numbers and differential together with platelets forms part of the basic assessment of the FBC. All of the results have to be interpreted in the context of the age, sex and clinical circumstances of the individual patient.

Figure 7.1 shows how the MCV may be of value in subdividing the anaemias into major subgroups.

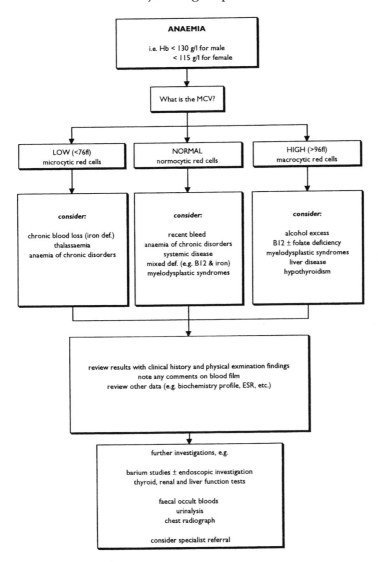

Fig. 7.1   Simple algorithm for classification and investigation of anaemia based on the MCV

Anaemia of chronic disorders

Typical features of this anaemia include the following:

1. The MCV is usually normal or moderately reduced. Occasionally indices may be identical to those found in iron deficiency.
2. The anaemia is of mild to moderate severity and usually non-progressive.
3. Serum ferritin is usually normal but may be raised.
4. Serum iron and TIBC are normal or reduced.
5. Bone marrow iron stores are plentiful.

Chronic disorder anaemia is found in chronic inflammatory diseases, e.g. chronic infection, stasis ulceration, bacterial endo-carditis, tuberculosis, collagen disorder, rheumatoid arthritis, SLE, other connective tissue disorders, sarcoid, malignancy, in the presence of carcinoma and lymphoma but not necessarily indicating marrow involvement.

The anaemia of chronic disorders comprises a major group of anaemias. It is not a haematinic deficiency. Instead there is impaired utilization of iron and studies suggest the marrow is less responsive to erythropoietin. There is also a lower than expected rise in erythropoietin, suggesting some inhibition in its pathway. In some inflammatory states elevated levels of IL-1 have been identified. IL-1 has been shown *in vitro* to inhibit erythroid colony formation. Detailed studies suggest a synergistic effect of IL-1 and T cells to produce interferon-γ which is capable of suppressing erythroid activity. In inflammatory states there may also be elevated levels of TNF and this also seems to have an inhibitory effect on erythropoiesis mediated by the release of interferon-β from marrow stromal cells.

Most secondary anaemias do not require therapy. Where patients have significant symptoms, supportive transfusion can be given. Erythropoietin may produce responses in secondary anaemias but the need for and benefit of a response to erythropoietin are not established. The use of erythropoietin in chronic disorder anaemia cannot be considered as standard management.

Haemolytic anaemias

This term refers to anaemia resulting from reduced red blood cell survival. There are many causes, including abnormalities of the red cell membrane, abnormalities of the Hb molecule and red cell enzyme disorders. Although complex, these all have one feature in common: *shortened red blood cell life span.*

At the end of their functional life (90-120 days), red blood cells are removed from the circulation by the reticuloendothelial system (macrophages in marrow, liver and spleen). Effete red cells are replaced by new red cells which enter the circulation from the marrow. Normally the number of cells removed is equivalent to those entering the circulation. If, however, an excess of cells is removed from the blood, the condition termed haemolytic anaemia occurs. In effect, this is an exaggeration of the normal process of cell renewal and replacement. The haemolytic anaemias are a complex group of disorders that arise through a variety of defects, either inherited (i.e. they have a genetic basis) or acquired through drugs or infection.

There are three basic abnormalities that lead to haemolytic anaemia and these are:

1. Abnormalities of the Hb molecule, for example, sickle cell anaemia (see slide question 17; data interpretation question 10);
2. Disorders resulting in reduced red cell life span due to defects in the red cell membrane making them more likely to be subjected to early removal by the scavenging system, e.g. hereditary spherocytosis (see data interpretation questions 18 and 21);
3. Red cell enzyme abnormalities, for example G6PD deficiency (see data interpretation question 2).

Red cell housekeeping functions

The red cell, itself, may conveniently be considered as existing solely for the transport of Hb and hence oxygen. Red cells possess a unique, highly flexible biconcave disc structure that is able to traverse the narrow capillaries of the microcirculation and the splenic sinuses. In order to maintain the integrity of its cellular membrane the red cell remains metabolically active throughout its life. During maturation the red cell loses its nucleus and most of its cytoplasmic organelles and therefore is unable to synthesize proteins such as enzymes. The mature red cell therefore contains a finite amount of enzymes and has no potential for renewal.

It has been suggested that the red cell must travel through 500 km of blood vessel during its life and during that time it will be required to withstand the force of cardiac contraction more than half a million times. It is not surprising that defects in red cell structure, or in the ability to maintain that structure because of metabolic defects, lead to shortened red cell life span and haemolytic anaemia.

Red cells, although lacking a nucleus, are not simply passive bags containing Hb. Instead, these cells are responsible for maintaining their own integrity by generating energy-rich compounds such as ATP and NADP from the breakdown of glucose molecules via the glycolytic (Embden–Meyerhof) pathway and hexose monophosphate shunt. Red cells need to maintain their cytoskeleton intact in order to allow efficient transfer of oxygen and carbon dioxide. To do this the red cell must retain its biconcave disc shape, an activity which is, in part, carried out by ATP-dependent enzymes and glutathione. Glutathione is a sulphur-containing molecule that exists in an oxidized (GSSG) and reduced (G-SH) form. After oxidation the reduced form of glutathione is generated via the hexose monophosphate shunt. A constant supply of glutathione is required to allow repair of oxidative damage to red cell membranes and Hb molecules.

General features of excessive red cell breakdown

Although the diseases differ in their cause, there are many features common to the haemolytic anaemias which are of some diagnostic help when faced with a patient in whom haemolysis is suspected.

Laboratory tests available for the investigation of haemolytic anaemias

Peripheral blood count

The automated blood count provides much useful information and, apart from measuring Hb concentration, measurement of red cell size (MCV) and Hb content of the red cell (MCHC) are most useful.

Blood Film

Hereditary spherocytosis, elliptocytosis, acanthocytosis and stomatocytosis all have characteristic abnormalities. Other haemolytic anaemias may only have non-specific abnormalities such as polychromasia and are classified as non-spherocytic haemolytic anaemias and a red cell enzyme defect may be suspected.

Polychromasia, an increase in polychromatic red cells, reflects the presence of juvenile red cells which may be counted as reticulocytes. Examination of the blood film is very important in the diagnosis of haemolytic anaemia as it may be diagnostic or point the direction of further investigation.

Reticulocyte count

Reticulocytes are juvenile red cells which contain ribosomal remnants which are present for approximately the first 24 h. Appropriate staining will easily identify these cells, which can be counted either as a percentage of total red cells or expressed in absolute numbers. The number of reticulocytes in the blood is a relatively good measure of erythropoiesis and hence can be regarded as a measure of bone marrow response to haemolysis, whatever its cause.

Serum bilirubin

Serum bilirubin will be raised as a result of increased haemolysis. The hyperbilirubinaemia will be largely unconjugated. Increased excretion of conjugated bilirubin by the liver leads to increased stercobilinogen in the faeces and increased urobilinogen in the urine. The finding of a raised serum bilirubin and the presence of urobilinogen in the urine may be taken as indicating increased haemolysis.

Serum haptoglobin

Haptoglobin is present in the blood to bind free haemoglobin, the haptoglobin-Hb complex being subsequently removed from the circulation by the reticuloendothelial system. Free Hb is only released during intravascular haemolysis. The finding of reduced or absent serum haptoglobin levels is evidence that recent intravascular haemolysis has occurred. Serum haptoglobins will be normal in hereditary haemolytic anaemias as the haemolysis is all extravascular (haemolysis occurring in the reticuloendothelial cells).

Red cell survival studies

Red cell life span can be measured by labelling patients' red cells with substances such as radioactive chromium, and commonly this measurement is combined with a determination of the major sites of red cell destruction by external counting with a gamma camera. The technique is time-consuming and takes at least 2 weeks to provide results and is not, therefore, a routine test. In haemolytic anaemia the cardinal feature is shortened red cell life span and therefore its measurement is restricted entirely to establishing that haemolytic anaemia is indeed occurring in situations where this is in doubt. No information can be gained about the cause of haemolytic anaemia.

Bone marrow examination

Bone marrow examination can demonstrate whether erythropoiesis is increased. Although this provides more direct evidence of marrow response to anaemia than the reticulocyte count, the information obtained is essentially similar. Bone marrow examination may also demonstrate the presence of an underlying low grade lymphoproliferative disorder (e.g. NHL or CLL), a well-recognized cause of autoimmune haemolytic anaemia.

Osmotic fragility

In this test the degree of red cell lysis caused by incubating red cells in sodium chloride solutions of various strengths is measured. Osmotic fragility curves are drawn for normal and test samples (see data interpretation question 18) and the MCF is calculated. This is the saline concentration at which 50% lysis occurs. Spherocytes will be lysed in stronger saline solutions than those required to lyse normal cells. In normal subjects the curve is steep and symmetrical, whereas in spherocytic anaemias the span and shape of the curve are altered and characteristically in hereditary spherocytosis a long tail of highly fragile cells will be seen. These abnormalities can be accentuated by incubating the blood for 24 h at 37°C prior to testing.

Refinements of this test have included the glycerol lysis time and acid glycerol lysis test which provide similar information to standard osmotic fragility tests. Whilst osmotic fragility is extremely useful in investigating haemolytic anaemias, it is important to remember that it will be abnormal in all cases of spherocytic anaemia whatever the cause. This is because hypotonic red cell lysis depends solely on the physical relationship between red cell surface area and volume. Osmotic fragility will be abnormal, therefore, in hereditary spherocytosis, some cases of hereditary elliptocytosis and acquired cases of spherocytic anaemia such as autoimmune haemolytic anaemia.

Heinz body test

The presence of denatured Hb in the red cell can be detected by specific staining techniques. The denatured globin collects in granules attached to the red cell membrane and, when stained, these are referred to as Heinz bodies. Heinz bodies will be detected where the Hb is unstable owing to an inherited defect, in G6PD deficiency or as a result of the action of oxidant drugs on the red cells.

The DAT

The DAT or DCT detects antibody on the surface of the red cell. The investigation of any case of spherocytic anaemia should always include this simple but informative test to exclude the diagnosis of autoimmune haemolytic anaemia before more complicated investigations are embarked upon.

Acidified serum test

The acidified serum or Ham's test is the commonest of a number of highly-specific tests for PNH. Although weak positive reactions are obtained in various dyserythropoietic states, strongly positive reactions are usually seen in PNH and this should not cause confusion. Its importance is that in any obscure haemolytic anaemia this relatively simple test should be performed to exclude the diagnosis of this extremely rare disorder.

G6PD screening tests

The fluorescent screening test is a rapid screening test for G6PD deficiency and should be performed before proceeding to quantitative assays. False-positive results may be obtained if the reticulocyte count is high or if there has been a recent blood transfusion.

Inherited haemolytic anaemias

Hereditary red cell membrane defects

The red cell membrane is a typical lipid bilayer which contains integral membrane proteins. Internally these integral proteins are bound to a protein cytoskeleton of hexagonal shape which is responsible for the maintenance of the shape and flexibility of the red cell. The principal cytoskeletal proteins identified are spectrin, ankyrin, actin and protein 4.1, of which spectrin is by far the most abundant. Hereditary spherocytosis and elliptocytosis represent a group of disorders in which there are deficiencies or dysfunction of these skeletal proteins.

It has long been recognized that these disorders are heterogeneous in that their clinical presentation may vary from asymptomatic to severely affected individuals; however, within families the degree of defect will remain similar in affected individuals. Studies of the structure and cytoskeletal protein content of red cells from affected members have demonstrated that the clinical heterogeneity of these disorders is reflected by the heterogeneity in the defects of the major red cell skeletal proteins. Although these discoveries have revealed much about the structure of the red cell membrane, they are not applicable to the routine assessment of hereditary red cell membrane deficiencies at the present time. The classical morphological features of the red cells on blood films determine their classification into hereditary spherocytosis, hereditary elliptocytosis, hereditary stomatocytosis or hereditary acanthocytosis.

Hereditary spherocytosis

Hereditary spherocytosis is a common cause of haemolytic anaemia and has a wide range of clinical and haematological expression. The characteristic abnormality is the presence of red cells with a smaller than normal surface area but a relatively normal volume.

The incidence of hereditary spherocytosis is of the order of 2 per 10 000 in people of European extraction and, although figures do not exist for other races, it certainly occurs in all human races. Males and females are equally affected and the pattern of inheritance is autosomal dominant. Only occasionally is hereditary spherocytosis diagnosed in patients in whose parents it cannot be detected by conventional laboratory methods.

Clinical features

Classically patients present with the triad of jaundice, anaemia and splenomegaly. A family history is important and it is necessary to enquire for family members who have had similar symptoms or who have had a splenectomy. Pigment gallstones are a common complication, although often they remain asymptomatic, whereas intractable leg ulceration is a rare complication. Although the diagnosis is commonly made in infancy, often the diagnosis may not be made until later life. In the neonatal period affected infants do not classically become severely jaundiced and, indeed, clinically obvious jaundice may not occur in affected individuals despite the occurrence of considerable haemolysis.

Splenectomy

Complete clinical remission is the almost universal result of splenectomy in hereditary spherocytosis and hence this dramatic response might even be regarded as a diagnostic hallmark of the disease. The anaemia is cured, the reticulocytosis virtually disappears and the serum bilirubin falls to the upper limit of the normal range. The underlying defect has not been cured, but the principal site of destruction has been removed. Spherocytosis will persist on the blood film along with the other classic blood changes that are due to splenectomy.

Blood picture

There will be anaemia of varying degree with normal white cell and platelet counts. The reticulocyte count will be raised 5–25% and considerable polychromasia will be seen on the blood film. The MCV is typically normal, although the MCHC is usually increased. The characteristic morphological abnormality of spherocytosis may be obvious but in mild cases may be difficult to appreciate.

Osmotic fragility

Osmotic fragility curves will usually be abnormal and the characteristic long tail of exceptionally fragile cells will be seen (see data interpretation question 18). Osmotic fragility curves may be particularly useful in the diagnosis of asymptomatic affected family members. In mild cases osmotic fragility curves may be equivocal, although the 24-h 37°C incubated sample may be more useful as the defect will be accentuated.

Differential diagnosis

The diagnosis of hereditary spherocytosis is not difficult if the following features are considered:

1. It is a haemolytic anaemia.
2. Spherocytes are present in the blood.
3. It is inherited in an autosomal pattern.

It is necessary to exclude autoimmune haemolysis by the DAT. In the neonatal period HDN due to ABO incompatibility is a spherocytic anaemia but for reasons that are not fully understood, the DAT may be negative. In this situation consideration of fetal, paternal and maternal blood groups and the presence of a potent haemolysin in the mother's serum will indicate whether this is a possibility and a family history will indicate if hereditary spherocytosis is likely. The diagnosis often cannot be made at this stage but will become clear if the spherocytosis persists beyond the first few weeks of life. At least one form of haemoglobinopathy, haemoglobin Köln, is a rare cause of spherocytic anaemia. In difficult cases this can be tested for by a Heinz body test and Hb electrophoresis.

Hereditary elliptocytosis

The presence of elliptocytic red cells in the blood is a relatively common finding worldwide and is the characteristic finding in hereditary elliptocytosis, a condition with a wider range of clinical and haematological manifestations than are seen in hereditary spherocytosis. The elliptocytes may, in fact, be elongated or oval in shape and constitute the majority of the red cells seen on blood films in distinction to the minor number (10-15%) of oval and elongated cells sometimes seen on normal blood films.

Autosomal dominant inheritance is seen in hereditary elliptocytosis. There are three major forms of the disease recognized:

1. Non-haemolytic hereditary elliptocytosis.
2. Haemolytic hereditary elliptocytosis.
3. South-east Asian hereditary ovalocytosis.

Glucose metabolism

Glucose is metabolized mainly via the Embden–Myerhof glycolytic pathway, which utilizes glucose in a series of steps which do not require oxygen. One mole of glucose generates 2 moles ATP, with lactate and pyruvate as the end-products of the pathway. NADH, required to maintain Hb in the ferrous form, is produced in the glycolytic pathway. About 10% of the glucose is metabolized in the hexose monophosphate shunt and results in the generation of NADPH, a cofactor required to maintain glutathione in its reduced form (Figure 7.2).

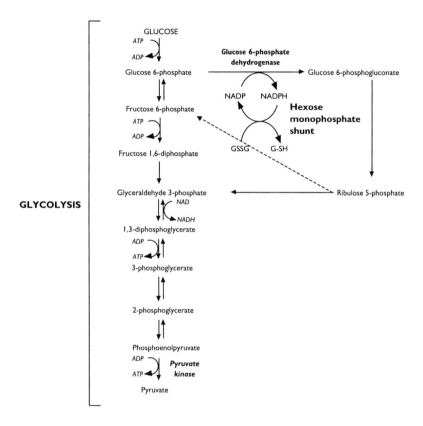

Fig. 7.2   Glucose metabolism: glycolytic pathway and hexose monophosphate shunt

G6PD deficiency

This is the commonest red cell enzyme defect leading to haemolytic anaemia; its role in the hexose monophosphate shunt is shown in Figure 7.2. It is inherited in an X-linked recessive manner; thus males are affected more frequently than females, although females who are heterozygous may still show features of the disorder. The condition is commonest in the tropics and subtropics and has become increasingly common in northern Europe, the UK, north and south America. The disease is extremely variable in terms of both its phenotype and genotype, with more than 300 variants now described.

Clinical features

Patients present with either a mild chronic haemolytic anaemia or are asymptomatic until there is oxidative 'stress' when NADPH becomes depleted and acute haemolytic crises occur. An acute haemolytic episode is typified by sudden onset of fever, malaise and abdominal pain coincident with jaundice and a fall in Hb concentration. Such stress conditions, by depleting NADPH, result in a fall in reduced glutathione which is required for detoxification of hydrogen peroxide produced by bacteria and certain drugs. Under these conditions Heinz bodies result from denaturation of Hb and the oxidation of membrane lipids leads to intravascular haemolysis. Conditions known to cause such crises include:

1. Fava bean ingestion (favism).
2. Drugs, especially antimalarials, sulphonamides, cotrimoxazole and aspirin.
3. Intercurrent infection.

In neonates G6PD deficiency results in a higher incidence of neonatal jaundice than in normal subjects. The aetiology of this is uncertain since a large proportion of neonates with G6PD deficiency do not develop neonatal jaundice.

Blood picture

Laboratory findings in patients with G6PD deficiency will depend on whether the patient has acute or chronic haemolysis. Patients with a chronic haemolytic anaemia will have a normochromic normocytic anaemia with a mild elevation of reticulocyte count, and only non-specific findings on the blood film.

Patients with acute haemolysis will have a falling Hb and marked elevation of the reticulocyte count. A leukocytosis is common. Examination of the peripheral blood will reveal spherocytes and Heinz body inclusions in the red cells. Biochemical testing will show an elevated serum bilirubin, reduced or absent serum haptoglobins and possibly evidence of renal impairment. Haemoglobinaemia and haemoglobinuria may occur if the attack is particularly severe.

Confirmatory tests

The G6PD fluorescent screening test is a useful test before proceeding to a quantitative assay. It must be remembered that reticulocytes contain higher levels of G6PD and, if the reticulocyte count is high, as it commonly is during acute haemolytic episodes or in the neonatal period, inappropriately high levels may be obtained. Reference ranges obtained in subjects with a similar level of reticulocytes can be used to resolve this problem. These tests are clearly not applicable if there has been a recent blood transfusion.

G6PD variants

Many of the G6PD variants examined by DNA analysis have shown alterations in the structural gene for G6PD due to point mutations. Three major forms of G6PD deficiency exist: G6PD A, G6PD A–, and G6PD Mediterranean. The first form is found in about 20% of American blacks and is a non-deficient variant due to a substitution (adenine to guanine) at nucleotide 376 resulting in a fast electrophoretic form of the enzyme. The G6PD A– mutation is present in African populations and about 10% of American blacks, and results from a double mutation, namely a valine to methionine switch at position 202 on top of a G6PD A variant, and is associated with a chronic haemolytic anaemia. The G6PD Mediterranean variant is the most severe form of the enzyme polymorphism found so far and is associated with acute haemolytic crises.

Hb disorders

Abnormalities in the structure of the Hb molecule or in the quantity of the various globin molecules in the red cells lead to a group of disorders termed the haemoglobinopathies. This complex group of conditions results in significant morbidity and mortality on a worldwide scale. Patients with these disorders are also seen in northern Europe and the UK, especially in areas with significant numbers of Greek, Italian, Afro-Caribbean and Asian populations.

Genetic control of Hb

Hb is made up of four protein subunits, each linked to a haem group. The subunits, however, are not identical but instead are two pairs of globin proteins whose production varies from embryo to adult to meet the particular environment at each stage.

Coordinating globin chain production

Different types of globin molecule are produced at varying stages of human development. After conception the human embryo develops and this produces three types of early Hb called haemo-globins Gower 1, Gower 2 and Portland. The structure of these molecules follows the same rules as all Hb molecules, namely two α-like globin molecules linked to two β-like globin molecules to produce the familiar tetrameric structure. Hb Gower 1 has two ζ (zeta) chains linked to two ε (epsilon) chains, i.e. $\zeta_2\varepsilon_2$; Gower 2 consists of two α chains linked to two ε chains ($\alpha_2\varepsilon_2$) and Portland results from the combination of two ζ chains linked to two γ (gamma) chains i.e. $\zeta_2\gamma_2$. These globin molecules are encoded by genes found on chromosomes 11 and 16 (Figure 7.3). The genes for all globins related to α-globin are found on chromosome 16 and the β-like globins are found on chromosome 11. This is because the α- and β-like globins have arisen from ancestral α and β-globin genes over many thousands of years.

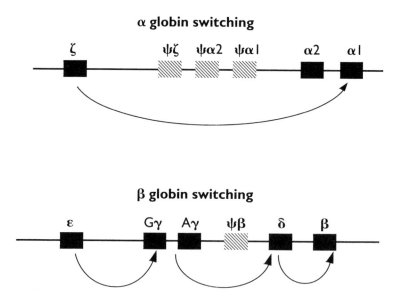

Fig. 7.3   α-like globin genes (chromosme 16) and β-like globin genes (chromo-some 11) showing physical location and sequence of expression during embryonic, fetal and adult life (see text for details)

Also of great interest is the finding that the order of these genes on the chromosomes reflects the order in which they are produced during development. Figure 7.3 illustrates the arrangement of α-like globin genes on chromosome 16 and the β-like globin genes on chromosome 11. From left to right, ζ is the first α-like globin to be produced in life. After ζ expression stops, α is switched on (so-called ζ → α switch). On chromosome 11 the arrangement of β-like globins follows the order (from left to right) ε → γ → δ → β, which mirrors the β-like globin chains produced during development. As the embryo develops into a fetus, production of ζ stops and α is produced instead. The α-globin combines with γ chains and produces $\alpha_2\gamma_2$ which is also called HbF. After birth γ chain production drops and both δ and β chains are produced. The main adult Hb is HbA ($\alpha_2\beta_2$) although a small amount of HbA$_2$ ($\alpha_2\delta_2$) and HbF is produced.

The mechanisms underlying the switch are, at least in part, physiological. We know that HbF ($\alpha_2\gamma_2$) binds oxygen much more tightly than adult Hb. This ensures adequate oxygen delivery to the developing fetus, which has to extract its oxygen from the mother's circulation. After birth the lungs expand, the oxygen is derived from the air the baby breathes and β chains are produced instead of γ, leading to an increase in adult Hb ($\alpha_2\beta_2$).

Hb abnormalities

These fall into two major groups: the first group of conditions results from alterations in the DNA coding for the globin protein. A mutation of a base (or bases) may lead to an abnormal amino acid in the globin molecule. In a protein like globin which is made up of 140 or so amino acids, one error would not be imagined to be of any great significance, but there are many examples of single base changes in DNA leading to marked abnormalities in the globin molecule which have serious clinical implications; these will be discussed later. The second group of haemoglobinopathies results from imbalanced globin chain production. The globins produced in these disorders are structurally normal but their relative amounts are incorrect and lead to the thalassaemias.

Abnormalities of globin protein structure

There are several haemoglobinopathies that are the result of an abnormality of the protein molecule. A well known example of this type of mutation is sickle cell disease, the commonest and most serious of the haemoglobinopathies. This disorder is caused by an abnormality of the β-globin molecule; the α chain is unaffected. The condition is found in Africa, some regions of Asia and parts of southern Europe, and is caused by a single base change in the β-globin gene. In the Afro-Caribbean population of the UK the gene is found in about 1 in 10 people. As a result of this mutation, an adenine in DNA is replaced by a thymine (i.e. A→T) which leads to an abnormal amino acid (valine) being substituted for the normal one (glutamic acid). This leads to production of the β^s (i.e. sickle β-globin) molecule. When red blood cells containing the sickle globin are under conditions where oxygenation falls the red cells elongate into sickle-shaped cells and lose their normal disc shape. The sickled cells do not flow well through small vessels and this leads to occlusion of these vessels and sickle cell crises.

Sickle cell anaemia   Patients with sickle cell anaemia are usually the offspring of parents who are both carriers of the β^s gene, i.e. they both have sickle cell trait, and homozygotes for the abnormal β^s gene demonstrate features of chronic red cell haemolysis. The red cells of these patients elongate into sickle forms when oxygen tension in the blood vessels drops, resulting in sickle cell crises.

Infancy   Sickle cell anaemia is often diagnosed before the age of 2 years. The reason sickle cell anaemia is not immediately apparent at birth is because the main Hb in early life is HbF ($\alpha_2\gamma_2$) which does not contain the β chain. It is only when γ chain production drops and β-globin production is switched on, that sickle cell anaemia becomes apparent.

Infective episodes   Bacterial and viral infections contribute significantly to the high morbidity and mortality in patients with sickle cell anaemia. One particular infection to which they are prone is pneumococcal septicaemia (due to *Streptococcus pneumoniae*). Other infecting organisms include meningococcus (*Neisseria meningitidis*), *Escherichia coli* and *Haemophilus influenzae*.

Dactylitis   The fingers and toes may become swollen and acutely tender because of small-vessel occlusion. Such episodes may be recurrent and result in permanent radiological changes in the bones of the hands and feet.

Infarction of the spleen   Severe pain may be experienced in the splenic area due to infarction of vessels within the spleen. The spleen may enlarge in early life but after many repeated infarcts may diminish greatly in size leaving only a small fibrous remnant. The function of the spleen is much reduced – a factor which may explain why pneumococcal infections are particularly serious in these patients.

Anaemia   Children and adults are often severely anaemic with Hb concentrations of the order of 6.0–9.0 g/dl. Symptoms of anaemia are less than expected for the degree of anaemia since sickle haemoglobin has reduced oxygen affinity (i.e. O_2 dissociation curve is shifted to the *right*), the anaemia is chronic and patients are well-adapted until an episode of decompensation such as that seen during an infective episode occurs.

Sickle crises   These episodes may be occlusive, aplastic or haemolytic. In the occlusive form patients complain of severe bone and abdominal pain. Bone pain is often felt in the long bones and spine and is due to occlusion of small vessels. Often these attacks are brought on by infection or dehydration, although in many cases no obvious cause is found. Aplastic crises are manifested by a sudden reduction in marrow function, usually in the red cells predominantly. In many cases a viral cause such as parvovirus infection is implicated. In most cases the aplastic phase is self-limited and after a week or two the marrow begins to function normally again.

Leg ulcers   In many haemoglobinopathies, including sickle cell anaemia, chronic ischaemic leg ulceration is found. This may improve with blood transfusion, which enhances tissue oxygenation.

Other problems   These include priapism in males (sustained painful penile erection), avascular necrosis of the head of the femur or humerus, arthritis and osteomyelitis; (the latter is due predominantly to *Salmonella* infection).

Diagnosis   Anaemia, as mentioned earlier, is usual in patients with sickle cell anaemia. The Hb may be between 6.0 and 9.0 g/dl, although in many cases it may be much lower. The red cell indices, including MCV and MCH, are normal. Examination of the blood film shows marked variation in red cell size with prominent sickle cells. Reticulocytes may be elevated reflecting intense bone marrow production of red cells. Biochemistry tests will often reveal raised serum bilirubin due to excess red cell breakdown.

Confirmatory tests   As with all disorders, a thorough history should be taken, which may reveal a positive family history or a past history of crises. Hb electrophoresis, which is a technique for separating Hb on a gel using electric current, will show mainly sickle Hb ($\alpha_2\beta^s_2$) with no normal Hb A ($\alpha_2\beta_2$). HbF ($\alpha_2\gamma_2$) may be elevated to about 20% of total Hb.

Management   Early and effective treatment of crises is essential and is best carried out in hospital. Intravenous fluids should be given since most patients are usually dehydrated because of poor oral intake of fluid and also excessive loss due to fever. Antibiotics should be given if infection is suspected before culture results from blood, urine or sputum are reported. Analgesia will often be required. In many cases i.v. opiates such as pethidine will be required, especially when patients are first admitted to hospital. This can later be changed to oral medication after the initial crisis is dealt with and under control.

   Between attacks patients should be treated with long-term prophylactic penicillin. Haematinic replacement will be required in the form of folic acid since patients become folate-depleted, continuous chronic haemolysis leading to eventual exhaustion of body stores.

Sickle cell trait   These asymptomatic carriers possess one abnormal β^s gene and one normal β gene. The blood film is usually normal and neither the FBC nor film can be used for diagnostic purposes. Detection of the carrier state relies on Hb electrophoresis.

The thalassaemias

This group of haemoglobinopathies arises as a result of diminished or absent production of one or more globin chains. In α-thalassaemia there is a relative lack of α-globin and an excess of β-globin. The net result is imbalanced globin chain production. The thalassaemias are the commonest single-gene disorders worldwide, occurring at high frequency in the Mediterranean, Middle East, India and Asia. In common with some other Hb disorders, α-thalassaemia is found in high frequency in areas where malaria is endemic and appears to offer some protection against this parasite. This selection pressure keeps the gene frequency for these serious disorders at a high level.

Thalassaemias are named after the gene affected; in α-thalassaemia the α-globin gene is altered in such a way that either reduced α-globin synthesis occurs or α-globin is absent from red cells. Various degrees of severity of thalassaemia are found and these reflect the type of mutation or deletion of the α or β-globin gene.

α-Thalassaemia

There are two α-globin genes on chromosome 16. Since there are two copies of each chromosome, there are a total of four α-globin genes per cell. Like sickle cell anaemia, described earlier, patients can either have mild α-thalassaemia (α-thalassaemia trait) where one or two α-globin genes are affected, or may have severe α-thalassaemia if three or four of the genes are affected. Thalassaemias such as α-thalassaemia may be the result of small mutations in the α-globin gene or, more commonly, a large deletion of the whole α-globin complex occurs. The normal person is described as αα/αα, meaning that he or she has normal copies of all four α-globin genes. A silent carrier results from loss of one α-globin gene (–α/αα). α-Thalassaemia minor is the result of loss of two α-globin genes from one chromosome (– –/αα or –α/–α). Such a patient will have mild anaemia. A severely affected person may have only one α-globin gene (– –/–α) and is termed as α-thalassaemia major (HbH disease). Loss of all four α-globin genes (– –/– –) results in death *in utero* (hydrops fetalis) since the fetus can only make Hb Bart's consisting of four γ chains (γ_4) instead of HbF ($\alpha_2\gamma_2$).

β-Thalassaemia

Unlike α-globin, of which there are four copies per cell, there are only two copies of the β-globin gene. An abnormality in one β-globin gene leads to β-thalassaemia trait and if the abnormality affects both copies, the patient has β-thalassaemia major. In contrast to α-thalassaemia, most β-thalassaemias are due to single point mutations (rather than large deletions) in the β-globin gene. In β-thalassaemia, where both β genes are affected, patients have severe anaemia requiring lifelong support with blood transfusions. Patients subsequently have problems with iron overload. The marrow attempts to make red cells but erythropoiesis is ineffective with most red cells in the marrow never entering the blood. The condition is not obvious at birth because of the presence of HbF ($α_2γ_2$) but as γ chain production diminishes and β-globin production increases, the effects of the mutation become obvious. The children fail to thrive or develop normally. They develop marked hepatosplenomegaly (due to production and removal of red cells by these organs). They tend to develop facial abnormalities as the flat bones of the skull attempt to produce red cells to overcome the genetic defect. Skull X-rays show 'hair-on-end' appearances, reflecting the intense marrow activity in the facial bones.

Investigation and management

β-thalassaemia trait   Hb may be reduced but it is not usually less than 10.0 g/dl. MCV is reduced to about 63–77 fl. Examination of the blood film reveals microcytic, hypochromic red cells. Numerous target cells may be present. Estimation of the Hb in the blood will show a raised level of HbA_2 ($α_2δ_2$), a useful diagnostic test in β-thalassaemia trait.

   Treatment is not usually required since these people are asymptomatic and are usually detected because of antenatal tests or on routine blood count, for example preoperatively.

β-thalassaemia major   These are the homozygous patients with two copies of the abnormal β-thalassaemia gene. The condition is severe and death in childhood occurs due to severe anaemia unless regular transfusions are carried out. The blood picture shows severe anaemia with Hb levels around 3.0–9.0 g/dl. The cells are very abnormal morphologically and show marked variation in size and shape; target cells and nucleated red cells are seen. Staining of red cells with methyl violet will show red cell inclusions; these contain precipitated α globin.

Hb electrophoresis will show mainly HbF ($\alpha_2\gamma_2$). In some β-thalassaemias there may be a little HbA ($\alpha_2\beta_2$) if some β-globin is produced.

Because of the severe anaemia, patients with β-thalassaemia major require lifelong blood transfusion every 5–10 weeks to allow normal growth and development in childhood and suppress endogenous erythropoiesis. These patients over-absorb iron and develop iron overload. Desferrioxamine is used to reduce the degree of iron overload. This is given subcutaneously for about 12 h a day for 5 days of the week and causes iron to be excreted in the urine and the stool. Splenectomy may be required especially if the spleen is massive but is avoided until after the age of 5 years because of the increased risk of infection. Infective episodes should be treated promptly and effectively with i.v. antibiotics.

α-thalassaemia minor   This is the asymptomatic carrier state and may be recognized once other causes of microcytic anaemia are excluded (for example, iron deficiency). No therapy is required for this condition.

HbH disease (– –/– α)   Here only one copy of the α-globin gene is functioning. Moderate anaemia is found with a Hb of around 8.0–9.0 g/dl. Mild jaundice (reflecting haemolysis) may be present. Infection, drug treatment and pregnancy may worsen the anaemia.

The blood film shows red cell abnormalities, including hypochromia, target cells, nucleated red cells and increased reticulocytes. Using the stain brilliant cresyl blue, so-called HbH inclusions may be seen. These represent tetramers of β-globin (β_4) that have polymerized due to the relative lack of α chains. The haemoglobin pattern in these patients consists of 2–40% HbH (β_4) along with some HbA, A_2 and F. Treatment is not usually required, although prompt treatment of infection is advisable. Folic acid supplements should be given, especially in patients who are pregnant. Splenectomy has been shown to be of benefit in some patients with HbH disease.

Hb Bart's hydrops fetalis (– –/– –)   In this state, where all four α-globin genes are affected, only γ chains are produced. These form tetramers (γ_4) which bind oxygen very tightly and so tissue oxygenation falls. This happens because Hb Bart's will not give up oxygen to the tissues that require it. These fetuses are either still-born or die soon after birth. They are pale, distended, jaundiced and have marked hepatosplenomegaly and ascites. Their Hb is around 6.0 g/dl and the film is very abnormal with hypochromic red cells, target cells, increased reticulocytes and nucleated red cells. Hb analysis shows mainly Hb Bart's (γ_4) with a small amount of HbH (β_4); HbA, A_2 and F are absent.

Advances in the management of globin disorders

Diseases such as thalassaemia major are currently treated by suppressing the underlying ineffective haematopoiesis using a hypertransfusion programme supported by iron chelation therapy. When used early in the disease the disfiguring bone expansion characteristic of the disease as well as other sequelae are avoided. However, the hypertransfusion regimens have been in use now for about 20 years and, although largely effective, are cumbersome and have low compliance rates. Novel therapies are sought that may make the management of thalassaemias and other Hb disorders more straightforward. Three areas of development are promising: the upregulation of HbF, bone marrow transplantation and gene therapy.

Manipulation of HbF

Adult Hb comprises HbA ($\alpha_2\beta_2$) which makes up the majority of Hb, along with HbA$_2$ ($\alpha_2\delta_2$). During embryonic and fetal development both α-like (ζ, α_1 and α_2) and β-like (ϵ, Gγ, Aγ, δ and β) chains are transcribed in a well-defined and orderly sequence (Figure 7.4). β-globin gene expression increases during the third trimester and the final switch from γ to β and δ (i.e. HbA and HbA$_2$) occurs around the time of birth. The control of the switching of different Hb genes is not fully understood but appears to involve erythroid lineage transcription factors with cis-acting regulatory DNA sequences. These sequences are located in the globin gene promoters, in enhancers 3' (i.e. downstream) to β and γ genes.

It has been recognized for some time that elevated HbF levels ameliorate β-thalassaemia and sickle cell disease. HbF reduces HbS polymerization and so reduces sickling. Also, compound heterozygotes for the sickle gene and HPFH have no clinical manifestations when HbF is greater than 25% total Hb. It is uncertain what level of HbF is required in sickle cell disease to ameliorate symptoms but,

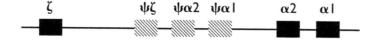

α-like genes on chromosome 16

ζ   ψζ   ψα2   ψα1   α2   α1

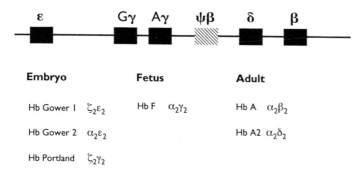

β-like genes on chromosome 11

ε   Gγ   Aγ   ψβ   δ   β

Embryo		Fetus		Adult	
Hb Gower 1	$\zeta_2\varepsilon_2$	Hb F	$\alpha_2\gamma_2$	Hb A	$\alpha_2\beta_2$
Hb Gower 2	$\alpha_2\varepsilon_2$			Hb A2	$\alpha_2\delta_2$
Hb Portland	$\zeta_2\gamma_2$				

Fig. 7.4 Globin gene switching (see Figure 7.3) during development allows the production of different embryonic, fetal and adult haemoglobins, which are listed above

from a variety of studies, an HbF level of greater than 10% reduces the episodes of aseptic necrosis; levels exceeding 20% HbF are associated with far fewer painful crises.

The goal has been to manipulate globin genes so that HbF levels are increased after birth. Certain disorders are associated with elevated HbF levels, e.g. acute haemolysis, phlebotomy, during recovery from transient erythroblastopenia of childhood and after BMT. In some species (e.g. baboons) HbF can be made to increase if the animals are subjected to acute erythropoietic stress. Several groups of drugs have been evaluated that have been shown to lead to increased HbF and these include 5-azacytidine, hydroxyurea and erythropoietin.

Drugs promoting the elevation of HbF

5-azacytidine.
Cytosine arabinoside.
Hydroxyurea.
Erythropoietin (rHuEPO).
Butyrate derivatives.

5-Azacytidine

This drug is an inhibitor of methyltransferase, the enzyme responsible for methylation of newly incorporated cytosines in DNA. It is
well-known that genes that are methylated show reduced transcription whilst those that are hypomethylated show increased
transcription. Therefore, by preventing the methylation of the
γ-globin gene, HbF may be increased. The drug has been shown to
be of value and does in fact increase HbF levels but it is only used
for patients with severe β-thalassaemia major because of the risks
of secondary cancers after prolonged use.

Hydroxyurea

Previous studies had shown that baboons treated with cytosine
arabinoside showed elevated HbF in reticulocytes. Hydroxyurea
produced similar results and has distinct advantages over other
cytotoxic drugs, e.g. low risk of secondary malignancy with
prolonged use. Hydroxyurea has been shown to increase HbF
levels in patients with sickle cell disease and has subsequently
been evaluated in a large number of clinical trials. Results in
β-thalassaemia major have been less impressive. The effects of
hydroxyurea are dose-dependent and the highest elevation of HbF
is seen at myelosuppressive doses.

Erythropoietin

In standard doses erythropoietin leads to an increase in HbF but it
has not, as yet, been widely used in the management of haemoglobinopathies. From cell culture and animal studies several
haematopoietic growth factors have been shown to elevate HbF;
these include IL-3, GM-CSF, and SCF. Based on these studies,
rHuEPO has been used in clinical trials and found to elevate the
percentage of HbF reticulocytes in patients with sickle cell anaemia
when given in high doses. There is some evidence to suggest that
rHuEPO provides an additive effect when alternated with

hydroxyurea. The dose required is fairly high at 1000–3000 i.u./kg 3 days per week, along with co-administration of iron supplements.

Short chain fatty acids

Butyrate analogues are known to be potent inducers of haematopoietic differentiation. There is evidence that elevated concentrations of butyrate and other fatty acids in diabetic mothers are responsible for the persistently elevated HbF in the neonates born to such mothers. Initial studies involving the use of butyrate to increase HbF levels in patients with sickle cell anaemia appeared promising but subsequent studies have been disappointing. One of the major drawbacks of butyrates is that the drug is required to be given as a continuous i.v. infusion. Experimental studies have also shown that, whilst butyrates may prevent silencing of a fetal globin gene, the drug cannot reactivate a previously silenced gene.

Bone marrow transplantation

In thalassaemia a large number of patients with severe thalassaemia have now undergone allogeneic BMT. The long-term disease free survival is 75% for patients undergoing HLA-identical allogeneic BMT. Three factors appear to be important in predicting the outcome of BMT in thalassaemia:

1. Degree of hepatomegaly.
2. Presence of portal fibrosis on liver biopsy.
3. The history of compliance with iron chelation therapy.

If no adverse prognostic factors are present, the overall survival of patients with thalassaemia undergoing allogeneic BMT is 95% with DFS of 87%.

In sickle cell disease a smaller number of patients have been transplanted to date. Unlike thalassaemia, patients with sickle cell disease do not require lifelong transfusion and iron chelation. Further, the mortality from sickle cell disease in the USA has dropped over recent years from 15% to 1%. There is therefore a less compelling argument for BMT in sickle cell disease.

Globin gene therapy

Red cells are an ideal target for gene transfer due to the ready accessibility of stem cells either in bone marrow harvests or peripheral blood during stem cell harvests. Most gene transfer programmes use retrovirus-mediated delivery of target genes to specific tissues. Globin gene transfer has been attempted with variable results. On some occasions the expression of the exogenous gene has been at levels too low to be of benefit to the patient. However, by manipulation of the regulatory elements (LCRs), higher levels of β-globin gene expression have been achieved.

Summary

Overall, there have been several significant advances in recent years and it is likely that manipulation of the patient's genes using a combination of agents, along with BMT for selected patients, will make the management of Hb disorders significantly better than at present. BMT, although curative, is more appropriate for thalassaemia than sickle cell disease, for the reasons stated above. We should be in a better position to judge the effects of these treatment strategies once more data are available from the various trials currently under way in the USA and Europe.

Raised Hb and polycythaemic states

Finding a male with a Hb >18.0 g/dl or a female with a level of >16.5 g/dl raises the suspicion of polycythaemia. The haematocrit should also be considered in these cases: persistent elevation of the haematocrit (>0.51 l/l in a male and >0.48 l/l in a female) is suspicious. The clinical problem is to determine whether polycythaemia, a state of increased red cell mass, exists or not. It is usually possible to determine this by a systematic approach evaluating clinical and initial laboratory findings followed up by targeted further investigation.

The Hb and PCV alone do not reliably correlate with the red cell mass/volume. At massively raised haematocrit levels there is some correlation. Similarly, the Hb and FBC results do not reliably distinguish proliferative polycythaemia from other causes. The presence of red cell microcytosis, a leukocytosis with neutrophilia ± increased numbers of eosinophils and basophils and increased numbers of platelets may be present in primary proliferative polycythaemia; very high levels of Hb and haematocrit are usually associated with primary proliferative polycythaemia in the absence of underlying cyanotic conditions.

A review of the clinical history and findings should be the initial stage after finding a raised Hb and haematocrit. This should identify excessive smoking, diuretic therapy, recent high-altitude travel or high alcohol consumption as possible contributory factors. A history of pruritus after a warm bath or shower is very suspicious of proliferative polycythaemia. Physical examination should identify obvious abnormalities such as gross obesity, evidence of obstructive airways disease or cyanotic cardiac conditions. Hypertension may be present. The presence or absence of hepatosplenomegaly should be determined. Polycythaemic states can be classified as follows:

Polycythaemia due to autonomous marrow overactivity

A clonal neoplastic marrow disorder with red cell over-production independent of erythropoietin levels
PPP or polycythaemia rubra vera (PRV)

Polycythaemia due to erythropoietin-driven increase in red cell production

The secondary hypoxic polycythaemias:
causes include:
    chronic obstructive airways disease
    cyanotic congenital heart disease with right-to-left shunting
    high-altitude dwelling
    chronic alveolar hypoventilation, e.g. gross obesity, (Pickwickian syndrome)
    sleep apnoea syndromes
    altered Hb oxygen affinity, carboxyhaemoglobinaemia,
    high oxygen-affinity Hb abnormalities

Polycythaemia driven by pathological increase in erythropoietin production

Various renal lesions:
    polycystic kidneys
    renal neoplasm
    following renal transplantation
Other rare tumours:
    cerebellar haemangioblastoma
    uterine leiomyoma

Apparent polycythaemia - normal red cell mass, reduced plasma volume

May be transiently produced by diuretic therapy, dehydration, etc. When chronically present, suggests spurious polycythaemia or stress erythrocytosis (Gaisböck's syndrome)

Idiopathic erythrocytosis

Persistent elevation of red cell mass: no cause found but no clear evidence of myeloproliferative disease or PPP

Investigation in polycythaemia then follows a logical sequence: first to determine whether red cell mass is truly increased by carrying out isotopic red cell volume studies, and secondly, to determine the cause of the raised PCV. Red cell volume studies are carried out by isotope dilution methods using ^{51}Cr-labelled autologous red cells and ^{131}I-labelled albumin to measure plasma volume. An increase in the red cell mass of >25% of that predicted from nomograms is diagnostic of a polycythaemic condition.

Having ruled out obvious precipitating hypoxic causes, other possible contributory causes should be sought. This may include referring a patient for imaging techniques for renal, hepatic or pelvic pathology. More objective measures of chronic hypoxia may be needed, including blood-gas analysis, respiratory function tests and oxygen saturation monitoring.

Bone marrow aspiration and biopsy are not primarily helpful in the diagnosis of polycythaemia. Where the diagnosis appears likely to be PPP, bone marrow aspirate and trephine biopsy should be performed. Significant marrow abnormalities are usually present; these include increased cellularity, erythroid hyperplasia and a combination of megakaryocyte hyperplasia and dysplasia. Fibrotic changes may be present. Marrow histology is not always abnormal in PPP.

A raised level of B$_{12}$ is common in polycythaemia where there is an associated neutrophilia due to transcobalamin present in neutrophils. Clinical iron deficiency with a microcytosis and low ferritin are common findings in proliferative polycythaemia and may be present in some forms of secondary polycythaemia. Hyperuricaemia may be found due to increased cellular turnover. Assay of erythropoietin is available but is not yet part of routine laboratory investigation.

Management of secondary polycythaemia involves treating the primary cause. Where surgical intervention is required, e.g. to remove a renal lesion, the haematocrit should be corrected pre-operatively by venesection. Where the polycythaemia is a secondary response to hypoxia, it is usually best not to reduce the haematocrit actively since the increase in haematocrit is compensatory. In pseudopolycythaemia, correction of blood pressure, reduction of smoking and an avoidance of other stress factors usually results in an improvement in haematocrit.

Management of PPP involves normalizing the PCV as quickly and safely as possible and maintaining a target level of PCV, usually <0.44 in females and <0.48 in males. In milder cases this may be achieved by periodic venesection; most cases will require myelosuppressive therapy with hydroxyurea or radioactive phosphorus. The patient should also be advised to avoid dehydration. Long-term allopurinol may be necessary to correct hyperuricaemia and low-dose aspirin is probably advisable for the majority of cases.

Hydroxyurea is the most commonly used cytotoxic agent. Hydroxyurea has a fairly rapid onset of action and any overdosage can be quickly corrected by temporary withdrawal. Busulphan may also be used to control polycythaemia. This is an alkylating agent with a slower mode of onset and much slower reversibility. There is likely to be a longer-term leukaemogenic risk because of its action as a alkylating agent. Radioactive phosphorus is an established treatment and will produce a reduction in red cell mass some 6–12 weeks after injection. The potential for leukaemic transformation appears greatest with radioactive phosphorus and its use should be confined to those over 65 years at presentation. Other agents active in polycythaemia include anagrelide and interferon-α. Experience of the former in the UK is minimal; the latter is active but appears to have no advantage because of its expense, side-effects and route of administration.

> Monitoring of polycythaemia treatment is best done by checking the corrected haematocrit. The haematocrit/PCV produced from FBC analysers is derived from the indices measured. Within the normal range, the PCV is accurate. It does not entirely correct for trapped plasma; this becomes more significant as the MCV falls and the RCC rises. For this reason a spun haematocrit is preferable in the monitoring of these conditions, as it gives a more accurate reflection of actual PCV.

Idiopathic thrombocytopenic purpura

ITP is a common disorder affecting adults and children, resulting from the interaction of autoantibodies with platelet and/or megakaryocyte surface membranes. The overall effect is reduction in platelet survival due to peripheral destruction. ITP may be a coincidental finding on FBC examination or may present clinically with excessive bleeding, e.g. epistaxis, menorrhagia, easy bruising or gum bleeding. The platelet count may be in the range 10–100 × 10^9/l but can be lower than this at presentation.

After a firm diagnosis of ITP has been made (involving the demonstration of platelet-specific Igs and bone marrow examination, which demonstrates normal or raised numbers of mega-karyocytes, including an increase in young megakaryocytes) a decision about necessary therapy can be made. If the thrombocytopenia is mild (~ 20-50 × 10^9/l) and the patient gives no history of bruising or bleeding, a watching brief may be held with regular platelet counts since a rapid drop may necessitate the need for therapeutic intervention. In many cases, and especially in children, the platelet count will return to normal or remain in a safe range without requiring any specific treatment.

Therapy

Corticosteroids

These have long been the main therapy in ITP. The mechanisms underlying the effects of glucocorticoids are believed to include a diminution in production of the antiplatelet antibody. Secondly, the platelet-associated IgG may fall with a demonstrable rise in plasma antiplatelet antibody as the IgG is shed from the platelet surface. The third mechanism invoked is the interference with macrophage Fc receptors that aid in the removal of platelets from the circulation, shown by *in vitro* experiments. In the UK prednisolone is most commonly used in a dosage of 0.5–1 mg/kg body weight per day, as established by Dameshek in 1958, up to a dose of 60–100 mg daily. The initial high dosage should ideally be maintained until a response in the platelet count is seen (usually by 3 weeks) although long-term high dosage is undesirable. In 4 out of 5 adults treated, an initial response to high-dose prednisolone is seen within 1–2 weeks, after which the dose should be gradually reduced over weeks or months to a level which allows a safe platelet count. In a small proportion of patients the dose can be tapered off and a reasonable platelet count maintained after cessation of steroids. Other patients will require low-dose prednisolone or alternate-day steroids long-term.

IVIg infusion

This treatment is widely used in the management of ITP, including ITP occurring during pregnancy. Like steroids, the therapeutic actions are not completely understood but appear to involve the interference with clearance of IgG-coated platelets from the circulation and inhibition of macrophage function. IVIg administered at a dosage of 0.4 g/kg per day for 5 days has been shown to elevate the platelet count, although this effect is often transient. Intermittent doses of between 0.4 and 1.0 g/kg per day may therefore be required in a number of patients to maintain an adequate platelet count. An initial response is seen in 3 out of 4 patients, with substantial rises in the platelet count even if refractory to other therapies, and often the elevation of the platelet count is seen soon after starting treatment (within 1–4 days), with a peak rise between 7 and 15 days.

Danazol

This synthetic androgen/progesterone analogue has been shown to be of benefit used either alone or in combination with steroids in 30–40% of patients and may allow the steroid dosage to be reduced to an acceptable level. Side effects include masculinization of female patients, weight gain and occasionally hepatic toxicity. The usual dosage used in ITP is 200 mg three or four times daily for 1–3 months before tailing the dose off to 50–200 mg daily if a response is detected.

Immunosuppression

Because of the greater risks and number of side-effects of the immunosuppressive drugs, these are held in reserve for patients failing conventional treatment with steroids, danazol and splenectomy. Occasional patients may be unsuitable for steroid therapy (e.g. diabetes mellitus) or unfit for surgical intervention. Immunosuppressive drugs have been shown to be of some benefit to about one-quarter of adults with refractory ITP producing some improvement in the platelet count, although it may take 1–2 months before any benefit is detected. Immunosuppressive drugs used in ITP include cyclophosphamide and azathioprine. These act by reducing platelet-specific IgG production and their effects take weeks rather than days to be detected.

Other treatments

Plasma exchange has been used in the emergency treatment of ITP but, since much of the antiplatelet IgG is extravascular, the response seen is not usually dramatic. It may be considered in patients failing other treatments and in whom the thrombocytopenia is clinically deleterious. Colchicine has been reported to be of benefit in occasional patients. Similarly, there are anecdotal reports of occasional responses seen in patients treated with cyclosporin. Interferon-α has been reported to benefit a small number of patients with ITP secondary to hepatitis B and/or HIV infection and preliminary data from patients with refractory ITP without evidence of viral infection suggest some response.

Splenectomy

Although not a drug option, splenectomy is mentioned here since this procedure may be of considerable benefit to a number of patients with refractory ITP. Antibody-coated platelets are removed by the red pulp of the spleen and splenectomy should be considered in patients refractory to conventional drug treatment. Some 70–80% of patients with ITP respond to splenectomy and the rise in platelet count is durable in many cases. However, operative and postoperative risks, including pneumococcal and meningococcal sepsis, may be unacceptable to both patient and clinician.

ITP in pregnancy

Either corticosteroids or IVIg infusions are commonly used before delivery to elevate the platelet count above $100 \times 10^9/l$ and may be continued post-delivery to maintain a reasonable platelet count. Depending on the platelet count, a caesarean delivery may be preferred to conventional vaginal delivery because of the risks of haemorrhage during labour.

Gestational ITP

This describes thrombocytopenia occurring during pregnancy (analogous to gestational diabetes mellitus). This is more common than chronic ITP and is seen in 5–8% of all pregnancies. Of all women with thrombocytopenia at term only 2% will have true ITP. In gestational ITP the platelet count rarely falls to $<70 \times 10^9/l$ in late pregnancy. There is no previous history of ITP, antiplatelet antibody studies are negative and the platelet count normalizes after delivery. There are no extra hazards to the fetus and delivery should be managed on the basis of the known obstetric risks (cf. ITP).

Neutropenia

This is a reduction in the absolute neutrophil count to $<2.0 \times 10^9/1$. Neutropenia may reflect the presence of underlying pathology or may be constitutional in some populations. For example, Yemenite Jews and some African groups may have neutrophils as low as $1.0 \times 10^9/1$ with no apparent underlying pathology.

Causes of neutropenia

Drug-induced
Bone marrow infiltration
Benign familial neutropenia
Chronic idiopathic neutropenia
Isoimmune neutropenia
White cell margination
Infection
Post-infectious
Nutritional deficiency
Chronic benign neutropenia of childhood
Autoimmune neutropenia
Metabolic disease
Immunological abnormalities

Chronic idiopathic neutropenia

This disorder affects both children and adults and results in selective neutropenia with the haematological indices otherwise entirely normal. Examination of the marrow shows a selective reduction in granulocyte precursors.

Alloimmune neonatal neutropenia

This is the result of transplacental transfer of maternal antibodies (IgG) to neutrophil-specific antigens from the father, and present on the neutrophils of the fetus. The disorder affects 1 : 2000 neonates and the resultant neutropenia lasts for about 2–4 months before resolving.

Autoimmune neutropenia

Autoimmune neutropenia may be an isolated finding or may be secondary to other autoimmune diseases such as RA, SLE, Felty's syndrome (rheumatoid, splenomegaly and leukopenia), Hodgkin's disease, or related to immune mechanisms triggered by infection. The disorder may also be associated with ITP or auto-immune haemolytic anaemia. Antineutrophil antibodies (IgG or IgM) may be detected; immune complexes are present in some cases. As well as accelerated turnover of neutrophils, there is also impairment of neutrophil production in the marrow.

Congenital neutropenia syndromes

These include Kostmann's syndrome, an autosomal recessive disorder associated with otitis, gingivitis, pneumonia, peritonitis and bacteraemia. Patients present within the first year of life with neutrophil counts that are often $<0.2 \times 10^9/l$, mild splenomegaly and a marrow that shows gross reduction in mature neutrophils. Serum immunoglobulins and karyotype are normal.

There are several other syndromes associated with neutropenia – reticular dysgenesis, transcobalamin II deficiency, lazy leukocyte syndrome, Schwachman–Diamond syndrome, Chédiak–Higashi syndrome.

Cyclical neutropenia

This describes recurrent episodes (often 21 days) of severe neutropenia lasting between 3 and 6 days with aphthous ulcera-tion and lymphadenopathy. The disorder is a stem cell defect (as shown by animal models) and is best diagnosed by performing serial FBCs. Treatment with G-CSF, which shortens the neutropenic episodes, may be considered if the disorder is severe.

Drug-induced neutropenia

These include antithyroid agents (carbimazole), anticonvulsants, phenothiazines and NSAIDs.

Bone marrow infiltration and failure

Causes are numerous and include any metastatic cancer invading the marrow as well as leukaemias, lymphomas, myelofibrosis, MDS and megaloblastic anaemia.

Infective causes

These include hepatitis, HIV infection, typhoid, miliary tuberculosis and malaria. There is also increased neutrophil utilization in bacterial infection.

Immune-mediated neutropenia

This may be idiopathic autoimmune (i.e. analogous to ITP), alloimmune, or secondary to underlying connective tissue disorders such as rheumatoid or SLE.

Margination

Complement activation may cause acute and chronic neutropenia due to adherence and aggregation of neutrophils on endothelial membranes. A variety of causes have been identified including haemodialysis, oxygenators, burns and transfusion reactions.

Therapy

The principal concern with patients who are neutropenic is the increased susceptibility to infection which rises as the neutrophil count drops. The infection risk becomes significantly greater when the neutrophil count is $<0.5 \times 10^9/l$. Overall, the degree of neutropenia and likelihood of infection are dependent upon the underlying disease producing the neutropenia, such that neutropenia secondary to marrow hypoplasia (e.g. post-chemotherapy) carries a high risk of infection, whilst neutropenia secondary to chronic idiopathic neutropenia is associated with a lower infection risk.

The chronicity of the neutropenia has a bearing on the infective organisms seen; in acute neutropenia bacteria such as *Staphylococcus aureus*, *Pseudomonas aeruginosa*, *Escherichia coli* and *Klebsiella* spp. are common, while chronic neutropenia is associated with sinus infections, gingivitis, fungal infections but rarely bacterial septicaemia.

Investigation

This should include a carefully taken history with particular reference to drug administration. Patients should be examined for signs of bony tenderness, lymphadenopathy and splenomegaly. An FBC and film should be obtained looking for atypical lymphocytes or abnormal cells. A bone marrow may be carried out to detect abnormal infiltrates, hypoplasia, leukaemia, lymphoma or myelodysplastic condition. An autoimmune profile is useful for excluding collagen vascular disease. Antineutrophil antibodies may be detected in serum and viral serology may confirm recent EBV or another viral agent involved in the production of the neutropenic state (e.g. HIV). Haematinics should be checked in case the patient is suffering vitamin B_{12} or folate deficiency. B_{12} and/or folate deficiency are well-recognized causes of neutropenia. However, there is generally macrocytic anaemia and thrombocytopenia making the nutritional deficiencies relatively easy to detect.

Management

Many of the inflammatory signs of infection may be absent in neutropenic patients because of the inability to mount a neutrophil response. The main causal organisms are gut and skin bacteria and for this reason broad-spectrum antibiotics are used in an attempt to cover Gram-negative and Gram-positive organisms.

Many clinicians use prophylactic antibacterial and antifungal agents to reduce the number of serious infections associated with neutropenia. On occasions it may be justifiable to consider the use of G-CSF.

Acute leukaemia and myelodysplastic syndromes

In adult patients 70–80% of acute leukaemia cases are AML; the remainder are ALL.

The typical presenting symptoms and signs of acute leukaemia relate to manifestations of bone marrow failure. Patients commonly present with anaemia, infection or bleeding manifestations. Sometimes patients may be non-specifically unwell and abnormalities in the blood count lead to the underlying diagnosis. Disproportionately severe haemorrhagic manifestations suggest APML complicated by DIC. Gum infiltration and skin infiltration tend to be a feature of acute myelomonocytic leukaemias. In the acute myelomonocytic leukaemias very high WBCs may occasionally be found and the patients may have hyperviscosity due to leukostasis syndromes.

Leukaemia is a neoplastic process of bone marrow and diagnosis, therefore, rests on a demonstration of leukaemic blasts in bone marrow aspirate and/or trephine biopsy. Leukaemic cells are usually demonstrated in peripheral blood together with abnormalities in other cell lines. Circulating numbers of leukaemic cells need not be high. In fact, in the majority of leukaemia cases, the total WBC may be normal and in a small minority of cases leukaemic cells can be absent from peripheral blood.

Diagnostic classification of acute leukaemia is increasingly important. The initial distinction between lymphoblastic and myeloblastic leukaemia is critical since different drug treatments are involved. Further information from cell marker studies and cytogenetic analysis to supplement standard cytochemistry are now part of the standard diagnostic procedure in acute leukaemia and related conditions. Tests are summarized on page 270.

Morphology	Cell appearances on Romanowsky-stained blood films
Cytochemistry	Sudan black and myeloperoxidase will identify approximately 80% of AML
	Esterase stains assign monocytic cell lineage
	PAS stain – block positivity commonly seen in lymphoblastic leukaemias
Cytogenetic analysis	Specific chromosomal features:
	t(9;22) translocation (Philadelphia chromosome) seen in approximately 15% of adult acute lymphoblastic leukaemias and carries a very poor prognosis
	t(8;21) translocation associated with M2 AML sub-types. Younger patients; typically associated with good long-term survival after remission achieved
	t(15;17) associated with APML. The chromosomal translocation relates to retinoic acid α-gene. Association with disseminated intravascular coagulation at presentation. Responsiveness to All-trans retinoic acid. Carries a good prognosis once in remission
	inv(16) associated with a myelomonocytic sub-type, FAB M4, with an eosinophilia. Similarly carries good long-term survival prospects once in remission
	Monosomy 7 is usually associated with preceding myelodysplasia and signifies a poor long-term prognostic group
Cell markers	In acute myeloid leukaemia the phenotype CD13 and 33 are usually positive. Aberrant phenotypes may be identified with shared lymphoid and myeloid lineage
	In lymphoblastic leukaemia help characterize differentiation equivalent whether pre-B or T cell leukaemias. B cell ALL associated with a very poor prognosis

The specific molecular changes, apart from identifying sub-groups, also now create the potential for monitoring remission in marrows. Detection of minimal amounts of disease is possible; the clinical significance of 'minimal residual disease' remains to be determined.

Differential diagnosis

Clinical features of an acute leukaemia may overlap with severe aplastic anaemia and MDS. Diagnosis will be confirmed by information from peripheral blood and bone marrow tests.

Management of adult acute leukaemia

1. Confirmation of the diagnosis.
2. Supportive care.
3. Remission induction chemotherapy.
4. Post-remission consolidation therapy.

Supportive care in the acute leukaemias is vital. Prior to chemotherapy, the patient must receive appropriate treatment for active infection. Severe anaemia should be corrected by transfusion, except in the presence of extreme degrees of leukocytosis. Chemotherapy will produce lysis of the leukaemic cells and in situations of massive tumour load hyperuricaemia and renal failure may ensue unless the patient receives maximum hydration and alkalinization prior to starting therapy. The patient and family require counselling as to the significance of the diagnosis and the aims of therapy.

Chemotherapy

In AML combinations of anthracycline and cytosine arabinoside are the mainstay of chemotherapy. Additional drugs such as thioguanine or etoposide are usually involved. For ALL, remission induction therapy involves the use of vincristine and prednisolone together with an anthracycline and asparaginase. Soon after remission is achieved, prophylactic treatment of the CNS is undertaken.

In both AML and ALL chemotherapy will produce severe myelosuppression resulting in a period of transfusion dependency. The patient is at risk of bacterial and fungal infections. Patients are generally nursed in side rooms with or without the use of filtered air to minimize exposure to external pathogens. Carefully worked-out antibiotic protocols are employed for treatment of suspected infection. During remission induction patients may require transfusion of up to 7 units of red cells, 70–80 units of platelets and a period of up to 21 days on i.v. antibiotics. Management aims to support the patient through the course of chemotherapy and the ensuing 2–3 weeks of cytopenia.

Once remission is achieved, further chemotherapy is necessary to reduce the chances of relapse. In AML 2–4 courses of intensive chemotherapy are given after achieving remission. These consolidation courses of chemotherapy are as intense as the initial remission induction therapy, with consequent requirements for full supportive care. In ALL severely myelosuppressive therapy is given early on, followed by prophylaxis to the nervous system using a combination of intrathecal methotrexate and cranial irradiation. Thereafter, therapy involves maintenance for an 18-month period using 6-mercaptopurine daily together with weekly methotrexate. Vincristine and steroid courses are given at 3-monthly intervals.

The optimal number of consolidation courses for adults with AML is still not known. BMT has been carried out in patients who achieve remission. The optimum time of BMT has similarly not been determined. The UK Medical Research Council AML 12 trial seeks to determine more precisely the role of transplantation in the post-remission therapy of AML.

Available data show that bone marrow allografting has a greater ability to prevent relapse than chemotherapy or bone marrow autografting. This benefit is outweighed by the procedure-related mortality, resulting in equivalent long-term survival. Bone marrow allografting does appear to have an additional antileukaemic effect but procedure-related mortality appears to outweigh survival benefit. In the UK Medical Research Council AML 12 trial the use of BMT as a randomized option for the fourth or fifth course of therapy is being studied. In this trial a further development is the definition of 'good risk', 'standard risk' and 'poor risk' prognostic groups. Patients are classified as good risk if they have achieved remission after one course and have karyotypes such as t(8;21), t(15;16) and inversion 16. In these patients there appears to be no benefit from BMT; the chances of long-term remission with chemotherapy consolidation alone are very high.

Myelodysplastic syndromes

MDS are a range of acquired neoplastic conditions of the bone marrow. They present with features of marrow failure but bone marrow and peripheral blood features are short of the criteria required to make a diagnosis of acute leukaemia. Many myelo-dysplastic conditions do not progress; some will progress and ultimately become AML. Classification of myelodysplasia is shown in the table below.

Management of MDS consists basically of supportive therapy. The majority of MDS patients are in the elderly age group; the responsiveness to chemotherapy is not high. Patients with RAEB-t and others who proceed to AML may be treated with chemotherapy as for adult AML. A preceding MDS is an adverse prognostic feature. Younger patients with RAEB-t may legitimately be treated with AML protocols and/or considered for allogeneic BMT.

Cytogenetic analysis is a key part of the diagnostic assessment of MDS. As in AML, it may well assign independent prognostic groups which would benefit from more conservative or more aggressive strategies. For example, the identification of a 5q– abnormality which is common in myelodysplasia seems to be associated with a good long-term prognosis. Monosomy 7, on the other hand, identifies a group of patients with an adverse prognosis.

MDS FAB subtype	Marrow blasts (%)
RA	<5
RARS	<5
RAEB	5–20
RAEB-t	20–30
CMML	<20

>30% marrow blasts indicates progression to AML

Chronic lymphocytic leukaemia

CLL is the commonest adult leukaemia and is found mainly in the elderly. The median age at diagnosis is 65 years. Classical CLL is characterized by peripheral blood lymphocytosis made up of clonal B-lymphocytes with an essentially 'mature' appearance on conventionally stained blood films. A percentage of these cells are more friable and disrupt on blood film preparation, giving rise to 'smear' cells which can also be helpful to diagnosis. The majority of cases are asymptomatic. As disease progression occurs, complications of lymphadenopathy and hepatosplenomegaly occur due to lymphoid infiltration. Marrow function may be compromised as a result of infiltration, producing anaemia, neutropenia and thrombocytopenia. Occasionally, autoimmune phenomena occur and can give rise to warm antibody autoimmune haemolytic anaemia or autoimmune thrombocytopenia. In more advanced disease, immune function is compromised and an associated acquired hypogammaglobulinaemia is present.

The finding of a lymphocytosis in a middle-aged or elderly adult is most likely to be due to CLL. Film appearances are as described above. Immunophenotyping should be done and will show the CLL cells to express surface immunoglobulin weakly and to express the B cell surface markers CD19 and CD20, together with the aberrant expression of CD5, which is normally a T cell marker.

Cytogenetic and molecular studies are not part of routine clinical assessment in CLL. It is, however, clear from studies that approximately 50% of CLL cases have demonstrable cytogenetic abnormalities. These include trisomy 12, abnormalities of 13, 14q$^+$ and deletions of chromosome 11. Ultimately, these may be related to specific oncogenes or oncogene products and may eventually lead to the identification of specific prognostic groups. Karyotypic evolution may also indicate disease progression.

Clinical management involves confirming the diagnosis. Early cases with lymphocytosis only rarely require bone marrow examination. Cases with evidence of more advanced disease should have bone marrow biopsy as part of the staging. Patients who show diffuse marrow infiltration have a much poorer overall prognosis. Lymphadenopathy and hepatosplenomegaly should be documented.

Good supportive care is important. Patients with symptomatic disease should be made aware of their diagnosis and told to report infection symptoms promptly. They are immunocompromised with or without the added effects of hypogammaglobulinaemia, and symptomatic infection should be treated with antibiotics. A minority of patients with marked hypogammaglobulinaemia and recurrent infections may benefit from supportive immunoglobulin infusions.

Autoimmune complications should be managed with corticosteroids. Chemotherapy in CLL is reserved for patients with symptomatic or progressive disease. Chlorambucil, an alkylating agent, is still regarded as standard therapy. It may be given in a low-dose continuous form or intermittently until the disease is stabilized. Once stabilized, therapy should be discontinued, since long-term exposure to chlorambucil carries a risk of transformation to acute leukaemia or myelodysplasia. Steroids should not be given concurrently unless there are autoimmune complications. Persistent symptomatic lymphadenopathy may benefit from local irradiation. Occasionally patients with massive splenomegaly may benefit from splenectomy and should be prepared for the procedure in the normal manner (Pneumovax, etc.).

New therapies

Fludarabine and 2-CDA are new treatment approaches. They are nucleoside analogues but also seem able to induce apoptosis in CLL cells. Clinical experience shows that the response rate is greater and incidence of remission higher after exposure to these drugs but they do not appear curative and so far no data exist to suggest they improve long-term survival. Fludarabine is licensed as a second-line therapy for CLL and trials are under way looking at its use as primary treatment of the disease. Although well tolerated, nucleoside analogues are also myelosuppressive and are noted to produce a decrease in circulating $CD4^+$ cells with a potential risk of an opportunistic infection.

CLL is incurable. The median survival for most groups of patients is long, particularly in the early stages of the disorder. However, for a small number of younger patients life expectancy will be reduced by the presence of CLL. Approaches involving the use of fludarabine to produce remission followed by marrow or peripheral blood stem cell collection and high-dose chemotherapy are being evaluated. Similarly, the use of allogeneic BMT for the very small number of suitable CLL patients with an available donor is also being assessed. These complex and high-risk approaches should only be carried out at specialized centres and as part of ongoing clinical trials.

Staging systems

Staging systems give a measure of the status of disease at the time of treatment. They can also be used to document progression. The two accepted staging systems are tabulated, together with an indication of the median survival from diagnosis:

Rai staging in CLL		Median survival (years)
0	Lymphocytosis alone – low risk	14.5
I	Lymphocytosis + lymphadenopathy – intermediate risk	7.5
II	Lymphocytosis + spleen ± liver enlargement – intermediate risk	7.5
III	Lymphocytosis + anaemia (Hb 11.0 g/dl) – high risk	2.5
IV	Lymphocytosis + thrombocytopenia (platelets <100 × 10^9/l not due to autoimmune effects) – high risk	2.5
Binet staging system		
A	Lymphocytosis + <3 areas of lymphadenopathy	14
B	Lymphocytosis + ≥ 3 areas of lymphadenopathy	5
C	Compromised marrow function – anaemia, thrombocytopenia + A or B above	2.5

CLL variants

Lymphoma/leukaemia syndrome

In low- and intermediate-grade lymphomas, circulating lymphoid cells may be present at certain phases of the disease. Morphology may vary in blood films; surface marker analysis will usually show these cells to differ significantly from classical CLL.

Prolymphocytic leukaemia is a CLL syndrome characterized by massive splenomegaly and often very high lymphocyte counts up to 400 × 10^9/l. The cells have characteristic morphology with prominent nucleoli. The cells express surface immunoglobulin very strongly.

HCL presents with circulating atypical lymphocytes in low numbers and splenomegaly, together with neutropenia. Morphology is characteristic and hairy cells are B cells and typically express the FMC7 marker. Bone marrow appearances are characteristic. Management of HCL is supportive. Symptomatic cases will benefit from chemotherapy with 2-CDA or deoxycoformycin. Previously, HCL was treated by splenectomy and also showed good responsiveness to interferon-α.

Splenic lymphoma with villous lymphocytes is a disease of the elderly. The disorder is commonly confused with CLL but has distinctive morphological and immunophenotypic characteristics. Splenomegaly is common and may be massive, but lymphadenopathy is uncommon. FBC may show lymphocytosis and paraproteinaemia occurs in two-thirds of cases. The cells are positive for B cell markers (CD19, CD20 and CD22) as well as HLA class II and FMC7. SmIg expression is strong (cf. CLL where SmIg is weak). If treatment is required, this may take the form of splenectomy, splenic irradiation or oral chlorambucil.

Myeloma

There are approximately 2500 new cases of myeloma diagnosed each year in the UK. It is predominantly a disease of older individuals with a median age at presentation of around 65 years of age; fewer than 2% of patients with myeloma are under 40 years. The disease results from the effects of an incurable neoplastic clonal proliferation of plasma cells.

The principal clinical effects

1. The presence of a paraprotein–monoclonal IgG or IgA in 70–75% of cases. Monoclonal light chain production in serum or urine in 20–25%; 1% of cases are non-secretory. IgD and IgE myeloma are very rare. Associated with the disease is a reduction in normal immunoglobulins – so-called immune paresis.
2. Skeletal disease. Neoplastic plasma cells produce osteoclast-activating factor. In many symptomatic patients generalized bone pain and osteoporosis will be present at diagnosis. There may be loss of height and vertebral fractures in addition to the typical osteolytic lesions noted in up to 70% of patients.
3. Bone marrow suppression with anaemia resulting from infiltration of the marrow by plasma cells may be present. This can also cause leukopenia and thrombocytopenia. Associated renal impairment in some cases may worsen anaemia. Renal complications may be present in 20–25% of patients. They may result from dehydration and hypercalcaemia. Irreversible renal damage from light chain deposition occurs in a small percentage and is not ameliorated by chemotherapy and hydration.
4. Infection as a result of functional hypogammaglobulinaemia and/or neutropenia is a frequent presenting symptom, leading the clinician to suspect an underlying diagnosis of myeloma on the basis of this problem alone or associated with any of the above complications.

Type of complication	Clinicopathological contributory factor	Management approach
Infection	Hypogammaglobulinaemia Neutropenia Chemotherapy High-dose steroids	Patient and GP education Antibiotics (oral/i.v.) Prophylactic measures (Septrin, antifungals), IVIg
Bone pain/ fractures	Lytic lesions Osteoporosis	Analgesics, NSAIDs, Opiates Orthopaedic Local radiotherapy Chemotherapy Bisphosphonates
Hypercalcaemia	Reabsorption of calcium from bones (osteoclast- activating factor)	Hydration, loop diuretics (e.g. frusemide) Corticosteroids Bisphosphonates (i.v. pamidronate) Chemotherapy
Renal	Dehydration Hypercalcaemia Myeloma kidney Amyloid	Hydration ≥3 l/day intake Chemotherapy Other supportive treatment, including dialysis
Hyperviscosity	High paraprotein levels Polymerizing immunoglobulin molecules	Hydration, plasmapheresis, plasma exchange Chemotherapy
Spinal compression	Spinal deposits, vertebral collapse	Early diagnosis MRI scanning/CT scanning Dexamethasone Local radiotherapy Rehabilitation
Neuropathy	Light chain neurological damage	Supportive treatment Chemotherapy Plasma exchange
Anaemia	Marrow infiltration Renal impairment Haemodilution	Treatment of principal contributory factors Chemotherapy Supportive transfusion Erythopoietin
Depression/ anxiety	One or more of above General uncertainty about future management approaches	Awareness of problem Social and psychological support

Patients with myeloma and plasma cell neoplasms occasionally present as neurological emergencies due to solitary plasmacytoma deposits causing spinal compression. A range of the clinical complications, contributory factors and management approaches is tabulated.

Supportive therapy focusing on the clinical complications and, wherever possible, their early treatment and/or prevention is fundamental. The condition appears intrinsically incurable with existing treatment approaches. During the last decade a range of therapeutic options has emerged, including high-dose chemotherapy and peripheral blood stem cell or bone marrow transplantation.

For the majority of older myeloma patients (>70 years) there are no convincing data to suggest alternatives to regular pulses of oral melphalan ± prednisolone. These are given at 4–6 weekly intervals to stabilize the disease – the so-called plateau phase. Once in plateau such patients are best left off treatment until such time as further disease progression occurs. Survival is not increased by continued chemotherapy and morbidity from infection and secondary myelodysplasia may be increased.

For younger myeloma patients there remains debate as to whether combinations of chemotherapy, including the use of nitrosoureas and anthracyclines, produce better survival than melphalan ± prednisolone as given for the elderly. Published literature shows many trials when there is no apparent advantage; the UK Medical Research Council 6th Myeloma Study did show a significant advantage for a combination treatment involving alternating cycles of Adriamycin and BCNU with oral cyclophosphamide and melphalan. Combination chemotherapy is given in an equivalent fashion to melphalan to produce a plateau of the disease characterized by a stable level of paraprotein and absence of progressive symptoms.

The discovery that high doses of dexamethasone combined with infusion of vincristine and Adriamycin produced remarkable responses in relapsed and refractory patients led to studies involving this combination of treatment as front-line approach. While response is more rapid and the degrees of responsiveness are greater, this therapy does not produce any increase in survival. It is generally more complex to administer requiring the use of a central indwelling i.v. line and associated risks. Following this therapy up with high-dose chemotherapy using melphalan ± rescue with peripheral blood stem cells or bone marrow will produce periods of long-term disease control off therapy, but as yet no clear data have emerged to suggest that this approach increases survival. It is certainly true, however, that where patients achieve complete remission there appears much more scope for reduction in complications associated with the disease, particularly progression of bony disease. Such approaches are being evaluated in various clinical trials. Important end-points in the analysis of these trials will be the duration and quality of survival from such approaches.

Allogeneic BMT has been carried out in myeloma. A small number of patients do appear to benefit but the approach is not applicable to the vast majority of myeloma patients.

Data on the use of interferon-α as therapy after achievement of plateau phase in myeloma suggest that this period can be prolonged by such maintenance therapy. Survival, however, does not appear to be increased. There are also promising data to suggest that interferon-α given after high-dose chemotherapy may maintain the stability of the response. Data on this from larger-scale trials are eagerly awaited. It is certainly recommended that neither high-dose chemotherapy approaches nor interferon should be employed routinely except in the setting of clinical trials and studies where the data can be properly analysed and evaluated.

A disadvantage of conventional chemotherapy is that there is little impact on the progression of bony disease. The majority of myeloma patients will die from progressive, refractory myeloma, often with worsening of bony complications. Bisphosphonates, by inhibiting bone reabsorption, have been shown in clinical trials in Finland, the UK and the USA to reduce the rate of progression of bony disease and consequently the number of fractures and need for analgesia with their potential to alter the pattern of bony morbidity associated with the disease they appear to offer an interesting parallel approach for management of the condition.

All patients with myeloma will develop relapsed disease and ultimately become refractory. While a small number may legitimately be offered a high-dose chemotherapy approach, the majority will be managed with conventional approaches. Patients who relapse some time after achieving plateau are likely to achieve a second plateau with melphalan or simple combination treatments. The VAD approach described above will produce a high response rate but the survival may not be any different compared to the use of high-dose pulses of dexamethasone alone.

Radiotherapy is very helpful in palliating the symptoms of advanced bony disease, especially in relapsed and refractory patients. Radiotherapy should also be used early in the disorder for localized areas of bony pain which do not respond well to chemotherapy.

Prognostic factors of myeloma generally relate to its stage of disease and the presence of complications. Staging systems were originally devised on this basis. The Durie and Salmon system classified patients into low, intermediate and high tumour mass. Classification was based on the pre-transfusion presenting Hb, the level of circulating paraprotein and the number of bone lesions. Subsequent studies have shown the use of β_2-microglobulin as a valuable prognostic marker. β_2-Microglobulin is a peptide component of the class I HLA complex. It appears to be one of the single most important prognostic indicators; it can be corrected for renal impairment and still holds as a prognostic indicator. High levels of β_2-microglobulin are associated with a poor prognosis. A high proliferative index of plasma cells at presentation is also an adverse prognostic feature.

Splenectomy

Following splenectomy patients appear to be at increased risk from overwhelming septicaemia. The risk applies to capsulated organisms, particularly pneumococci. The effect results from loss of splenic function which plays a key role in optimal immune responses.

Elective splenectomy is a therapy for some haematological conditions. The reasons for splenectomy relate to hyperfunction of the organ, organ size causing pressure symptoms, the persistence of unexplained splenomegaly, or the procedure may be required for diagnosis. Splenectomy may have to be done as an emergency following trauma, spontaneous rupture or for anatomical reasons in complicated abdominal surgery. It is less frequently used as a staging procedure in Hodgkin's disease. Functional hyposplenism exists in sickle cell anaemia, some cases of essential thrombocythaemia and as a complication of coeliac disease. Following BMT with total body irradiation, patients are functionally hyposplenic.

Patients in all these categories are at risk of post-splenectomy infection. The nature of the risk is not quantifiable but prophylactic strategies are advised. Risks of infection are probably higher following splenectomy carried out for underlying haematological disorders. Where carried out for trauma, the risk exists, although it appears lower than for the former indication.

For elective splenectomy preoperative vaccination with pneumococcal vaccine would appear mandatory. On current guidelines patients should be re-vaccinated every 5 years; for those with poor antibody levels perhaps 3-yearly re-vaccination is advisable. *Haemophilus influenzae* vaccine should be given. Debate exists as to whether preoperative meningococcal vaccine is necessary as the immunity following this vaccination is short-lasting and only subtypes A and C are covered. Vaccinations should be given at least 2 weeks prior to splenectomy. If splenectomy has been carried out as an urgent procedure, pneumococcal vaccine should nevertheless be given postoperatively.

Patients undergoing splenectomy do have increased thrombotic risks. Active measures to prevent thromboembolism should be employed, including the use of antiembolism stockings and low-dose heparin anticoagulation. The use of anticoagulation may need to be adjusted depending on the haematological indications. Thrombocytosis can be expected to follow the majority of splenectomies and once the patient is discharged from hospital it seems reasonable to advise the use of low-dose aspirin for at least 3 months until the platelet count is settled.

There is a consensus that all patients should be advised to take oral prophylaxis with penicillin V 250 mg twice daily for life after splenectomy. However, there are no trial data to support whether this approach offers protection against pneumococci for all categories of patient. Previous guidelines suggested that antibiotic therapy should be given up to the age of 16–18 years. Debate has existed as to whether antibiotics should be given for 2 years, 5 years or life following splenectomy. Recently published guidelines suggest that lifelong antibiotic treatment should be recommended. However, not all patients comply. For patients allergic to penicillin an alternative such as oral erythromycin 250 mg b.d. should be offered.

Influenza immunization annually is advised and patients should be strongly encouraged to comply rigorously with advice on malarial prophylaxis. Hyposplenic individuals are at much greater risk of complications from *Plasmodium falciparum*.

As far as reducing the risk of fatality from overwhelming post-splenectomy infection is concerned, the most important procedure is to make the patient aware of the risk. They should have some means of identifying themselves as being at risk, for example, a Medic Alert disc or a card indicating that they lack a spleen. Antibiotic prophylaxis is not 100% effective and if they feel profoundly unwell they should be referred for medical attention urgently, most probably to their local Accident and Emergency Department.

Key points from the guidelines

1. All splenectomized patients should receive pneumococcal immunization. These should be carefully documented. *Haemophilus influenzae* type B vaccine is advisable. Influenza vaccination annually should be considered.
2. Lifelong prophylactic antibiotics are recommended. A decision to stop or not to proceed with lifelong antibiotics should be a joint doctor–patient decision.
3. Asplenic patients are at risk of severe malaria infection, notably *Plasmodium falciparum*.
4. Patients should be given a leaflet or card to alert health professionals to the risks.
5. Patients developing profound systemic symptoms with infection should be referred urgently for hospital assessment.

Reference

Working Party of the British Committee for Standards in Haematology. Clinical Haematology Task Force (1996). Guidelines for the prevention and treatment of infection in patients with an absent or dysfunctional spleen. *British Medical Journal* **312**: 430–434.

Some haematological indications for splenectomy

Lymphoproliferative diseases	Autoimmune complications, e.g. haemolysis or thrombocytopenia Organ size Therapeutic – HCL Diagnostic – CLL variants
Myeloproliferative disease	Myelofibrosis – to reduce transfusion requirements To reduce abdominal discomfort from massive splenic enlargement To reduce constitutional symptoms, e.g. weight loss and night sweats
Hereditary disorders	Homozygous β-thalassaemia – to reduce transfusion requirements Hereditary spherocytosis for recurrent, severe cases Pyruvate kinase deficiency Gaucher's disease type 1
Others	Autoimmune conditions: autoimmune haemolytic anaemia and ITP RA – Felty's syndrome.
Staging splenectomy	NHL and Hodgkin's disease – no longer a routine procedure

Modifying surgical blood losses

Most patients receiving blood transfusion are given allogeneic (i.e. donor) blood. Because of the risks in terms of both infection and immunomodulation there is renewed interest in reducing the quantity of such units transfused. Blood conservation will lead to reduced risk of viral infection and reduce chances of alloimmunization and transfusion reactions. Autologous blood (i.e. the patient's own blood) is useful when allogeneic blood is in short supply. Autologous transfusion is also of great benefit to patients who have antibodies to high-frequency antigens, e.g. anti-Kp^b, anti-H (in rare O-Bombay individuals) and anti-Vel. Jehovah's Witnesses may accept autologous blood provided it remains in continuity with their own circulatory system. Autologous blood reduces cross-matching by laboratory staff and may therefore reduce staff and consumable costs.

Minimising blood used for transfusion

There are several potential methods of reducing allogeneic blood transfusion:

1. Adherence to strict criteria.
2. Anaesthetic and pharmacological manoeuvres, e.g. hypotensive surgery.
3. Autologous transfusion through preoperative haemodilution, pre-deposit blood banking and red cell salvage.

Preoperative haemodilution

This implies reducing the Hb concentration prior to surgery with the aim of reducing viscosity, reducing red cell loss (through reduced haematocrit) and providing a bank of freshly collected autologous whole blood for return later.

Generally, 2–3 units of blood are collected with replacement using crystalloids or colloid solutions. The Hb is reduced to ~10 g/dl and haematocrit to 30% (0.3). Oxygen transport improves due to an increase in cardiac output. Haemodilution is probably safest in younger patients and those without pre-existing cardiopulmonary disease. Despite its use over the past few years, the clinical benefits in routine operative surgery are not well understood or accepted.

Autologous transfusion programmes

These may take the form of pre-deposit or salvage of red cells intra-operatively. This type of procedure is only of value in planned surgery and makes use of a well-established maximum surgical blood-ordering schedule.

Predeposit system

Patients deemed fit to donate and patients who are 'uncross-matchable' due to, for example, alloantibodies against high-frequency antigens should be considered for pre-deposit programmes. Eligibility varies but usually include Hb (needs to be 11 g/dl or greater) and age – elderly patients can tolerate pre-deposit provided cardiovascular assessment is performed and excludes serious disease; young adults and children are also eligible. Pregnancy poses particular problems and collection of units is unlikely to be of benefit in this setting. Donors with a history of epilepsy are not accepted because of the risk of seizures.

The procedure itself involves the collection of 2 units of blood: the first unit is collected 2 weeks before the operation and the second is taken 3–7 days prior to surgery. Iron replacement is usually given. Some pre-deposit programmes boost with rHuEPO enabling a larger number of units to be collected.

Laboratory testing of pre-deposited units

In the UK autologous units are treated identically to allogeneic units with full grouping, antibody screening and microbiological testing in case the autologous unit is transfused to the wrong recipient.

Blood salvage during surgery

Blood lost during surgery may be reinfused into patients using suction catheters and filtration systems. These techniques are expensive and not widely used in the UK at present. Two main methods are available:

1. Single-use disposable canisters (e.g. Solcotrans), where the patient is heparinized and anticoagulated blood is collected into ACD anticoagulant in the canister. Red cells are reinfused after filtration through a microaggregate filter.
2. Automated or semiautomated salvage (e.g. Hemonetics Cell Saver). Blood is collected, washed centrifugally, filtered and red cells are held for reinfusion.

Intraoperative autotransfusion has proved useful in cardiovascular surgery but may be used for almost any surgical procedure, provided there is no faecal contamination or risk of tumour dissemination. Red cells must be washed to remove tissue fragments and activated clotting factors.

Pharmacological agents and their role in reducing blood loss

Various drugs have been used to modify the coagulation and fibrinolytic systems. These include DDAVP, which improves platelet function. Platelet-inhibitory drugs, e.g. prostacyclin, have also been used. Aprotinin has been widely used in cardiovascular surgery, liver transplantation and other surgical procedures to reduce blood loss intraoperatively. Aprotinin also seems to have a platelet-sparing role during cardiac bypass surgery and the prolongation of the bleeding time is reduced.

Summary

There are several methods available for reducing the amount of allogeneic blood used during surgical procedures. For a variety of reasons (expense, lack of organizational facilities, cancellation of elective surgery, lack of trained personnel) these are not widely used in the UK. There is far greater interest at present in the USA where patients are particularly keen not to receive blood donated by paid donors with the attendant risks this brings. We will no doubt learn from the American experience and probably see these techniques used in the UK eventually.

Hypercoagulable states and recurrent thromboembolic disease

The coagulation system is a delicately balanced series of coagulation and fibrinolytic events. A defect or deficiency in one of the natural anticoagulants (e.g. protein C or S) will swing the balance towards thrombosis.

There are two principal types of hypercoagulable state: first, inherited, whereby the patient has a specific defect in one of the natural anticoagulant mechanisms, and second, acquired thrombophilia, which represents a heterogeneous group of disorders associated with an increased risk of thromboembolism.

Inherited

Inherited disorders associated with hypercoagulability

1. Antithrombin III deficiency.
2. Protein C deficiency.
3. Protein S deficiency.
4. APCR.
5. Dysfibrinogenaemias.
6. Dysplasminogenaemias.
7. Factor XII deficiency.

Patients under the age of 45 years evaluated for venous thrombosis have a prevalence of 15% for hereditary deficiencies of anti-thrombin III, protein C and protein S. These three deficiencies occur with roughly equal frequency.

Features suggestive of thrombophilia are:

1. Thrombosis at an early age.
2. Positive family history of thromboembolic disease.
3. Thrombosis at unusual sites.
4. Recurrent thromboembolism despite adequate treatment.
5. Warfarin-induced skin necrosis.

Thrombosis in thrombophilia tends to be venous rather than arterial.

Antithrombin deficiency

Antithrombin III is the major inhibitor of serine proteases and acts by inhibiting thrombin, IXa, Xa, XIa and XIIa. Antithrombin III is a glycoprotein of 50 kDa and is synthesized in the liver.

Antithrombin III deficiency was first reported in a Norwegian family in which the antithrombin III level was found to be about 40% of normal. The family had a history of recurrent thromboembolism. Inheritance of antithrombin III deficiency is autosomal dominant, thus the sexes are affected equally. The prevalence of antithrombin III deficiency in the general population is 1 : 350. Some 55% of patients with antithrombin III deficiency will experience venous thromboembolism at some time.

The predominant sites affected are the deep veins of the legs and mesenteric veins.

Type I deficiency represents diminished production of antithrombin III protein whilst type II is characterised by abnormal function of the molecule, although its concentration in plasma may be normal. Because of this, functional assays are preferred to immunological assays that provide an estimate of the concentration of molecules such as antithrombin III, proteins C and S.

Treatment

Intravenous heparin as standard therapy is used, although high levels may be required to achieve full anticoagulation (in view of the antithrombin III deficiency). Some patients may require exogenous antithrombin III administration in order to achieve anticoagulation with heparin.

For recurrent thrombosis long-term oral anticoagulation should be considered.

Protein C deficiency

Protein C is a vitamin K-dependent glycoprotein that acts as one of the major regulatory inhibitory proteins of the coagulation system. Protein C is activated to form activated protein C on endothelial surfaces by the thrombin thrombomodulin complex. Protein C acts as an anticoagulant by degrading activated factor V (Va) and VIII (VIIIa).

Protein C deficiency is inherited as an autosomal dominant. Affected heterozygotes have protein C levels of around 50%. The clinical features are identical to those of antithrombin III deficiency. Some 75% of affected individuals suffer venous thromboembolism. A minority will have non-haemorrhagic stroke. Onset of thromboembolism is in young adulthood, with the risk of thrombosis rising steadily with age. Warfarin-induced skin necrosis is more likely in patients with protein C deficiency.

Treatment

Standard anticoagulation, initially with i.v. heparin followed by oral warfarin, is used. Stanozolol and danazol have been shown to increase protein C levels in some patients.

Protein S deficiency

Protein S was isolated and characterized in Seattle (hence protein S). It is a non-enzymatic cofactor of activated protein C. Like protein C, protein S is a vitamin K-dependent protein and is synthesized by the liver, endothelial cells and it is also found in α granules of platelets.

Inherited protein S deficiency is autosomal dominant. The presentation is similar to antithrombin III and protein C deficiency. Clinical features are similar to those of antithrombin III and protein C deficiency. Skin necrosis is reported but is less common than with protein C deficiency.

Activated protein C resistance

Dahlback and workers described APCR in 1993 as a mechanism for recurrent thrombosis. He described patients whose plasma exhibited a poor response to activated protein C in an APTT assay. A defect in the factor V gene (Leiden mutation) was identified as the major cause. This point mutation occurs at the site at which activated protein C cleaves factor Va; this mutation makes the Va molecule biochemically resistant to inactivation by activated protein C and has been demonstrated in 20–40% of thrombotic patients and has a prevalence of 5% in the general population.

This may represent the commonest cause of inherited thrombophilia. Patients who co-inherit protein C deficiency are at greater risk of thrombosis than those who inherit protein C deficiency alone. In fact, APCR alone is probably not sufficient for the development of thrombosis and inheritance of other thrombotic risks or the presence of an acquired thrombophilia risk factor is necessary.

Dysfibrinogenaemias

There are fewer than 20 variant fibrinogens that have been reported to date that are associated with recurrent thrombosis.

Dyplasminogenaemias

Dysplasminogenaemias and hypoplasminogenaemias have been reported in 20 patients with recurrent thromboembolic disease.

Factor XII deficiency (Hageman factor)

FXII is the zymogen of a serine protease that initiates contact activation and the intrinsic pathway *in vitro*. Deficiency has been associated with a tendency to venous thrombosis.

Acquired disorders associated with hypercoagulable state

Pathological causes

Lupus anticoagulant syndrome.
Malignant disease.
Infusion of prothrombin complex concentrates.
Nephrotic syndrome.
Heparin-induced thrombocytopenia.
Thrombotic thrombocytopenic purpura.
Myeloproliferative diseases.
Paroxysmal nocturnal haemoglobinuria.
Hyperlipidaemia.
Diabetes mellitus.
Liver disease.
Homocystinuria.
Hyperviscosity.

Physiological causes

Pregnancy (especially postpartum).
Postoperative.
Immobilization.
Advancing age.
Obesity.

Lupus anticoagulant syndrome

This is due to an antibody (IgG or IgM or both) that prolongs the phospholipid-dependent clotting assay *in vitro*. The term is a misnomer since it occurs frequently in patients with no evidence of SLE and is seen in association with other autoimmune disease, drugs, infections, malignancy and in many normal subjects. Patients do not bleed unless there are other haemostatic defects present. There is a definite increased risk of both arterial and venous thrombosis. In recurrent cases the affected site tends to be the same.

Laboratory tests

The APTT is prolonged but is not corrected by the addition of normal plasma. The DRVVT and dilute thromboplastin test are useful screens for lupus anticoagulants.

Management

Patients are managed using standard regimens, including i.v. heparin initially followed by oral anticoagulation. Aspirin has also been shown to be of value in some studies.

Investigation of suspected thrombophilia

A variety of assays are carried out, grouped together as primary and secondary screens.

Primary screen

FBC.
PT.
APTT.
Thrombin time.
Reptilase time.
Fibrinogen concentration.
Liver enzymes.

Secondary screen

Antithrombin III assay.
    Functional.
    Immunological.
Protein C assay.
    Functional.
    Immunological.
Protein S assay.
    Functional.
    Immunological.
C4b binding assay.
Antiphospholipid antibody detection.
Activated protein C resistance.
    Clotting test.
    PCR (factor V Leiden mutation).

Of unproven value

Heparin cofactor II assay.
Euglobulin clot lysis time.
Plasminogen assay.
Tissue plasminogen activator.
Plasminogen activator inhibitor assay.

Applications of molecular biology to haematology

There have been several advances in molecular diagnostics over the past few years and most of these have found application within malignant disease, especially in haematology and oncology. These highly sophisticated investigations are used to confirm data provided by more conventional analyses or to aid in the diagnosis of difficult cases where conventional methodology has failed. Those techniques that are of most importance within haematology and general medicine are predominantly nucleic acid-based (DNA or RNA) and include:

1. Southern blotting and northern blotting.
2. PCR.
3. Cloning and sequencing of genes.
4. *In situ* hybridization.
5. FISH using specific gene probes.

These will be discussed in turn, with examples of their use.

Southern blotting

Southern blotting has been used since the mid 1970s, pioneered by Professor Ed Southern in Edinburgh. At the time, Southern analysis was seen as an improved method for mapping human genes and gave much higher resolution than conventional 'crosses' and standard genetic analysis. The method is extremely simple and elegant and requires genomic DNA as starting material. The technique relies on physical homology of a known fragment of DNA (i.e. the probe), allowing binding of the probe to its homologous sequence in the sample of digested patient or test DNA.

DNA is extracted from tissues and digested with bacterial nucleases termed restriction endonucleases. These enzymes cleave DNA at specific sequences, with each enzyme recognizing a different DNA sequence. After digestion of DNA, the fragments generated are separated on the basis of size using agarose gel electrophoresis. The smallest fragments will travel the furthest distance, whilst the large fragments will hardly travel any distance at all. The fragments are transferred to a nylon membrane and fixed permanently to the membrane using ultraviolet light.

Membranes are probed using specific (known) gene probes that are radioactively labelled; non-radioactive methods such as the digoxigenin system are now available as a safer alternative to radionuclides such as ^{32}P. The unbound probe is removed and the location of specific binding is detected by placing the membrane next to radiographic film. This is then developed using standard techniques and the autoradiograph generated will show bands corresponding to the position of binding of the labelled probe (Figure 7.5).

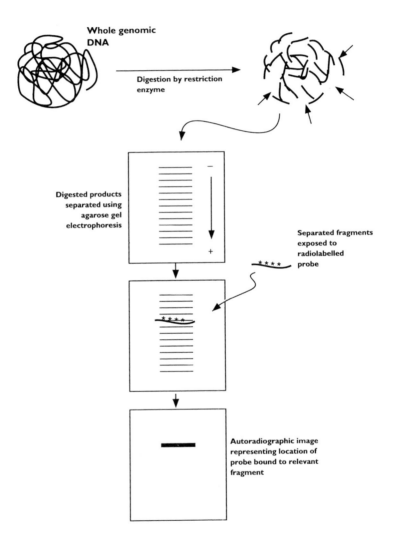

Fig. 7.5   Schematic diagram illustrating the technique of Southern blotting

It may not be immediately obvious how this information can help, but the size of the bands generated after digestion defines the configuration of the gene being investigated. To give one specific example, immunoglobulin genes undergo irreversible rearrangement during B-lymphocyte development. The reason for this is that immunoglobulin genes are present in the immature cells as non-contiguous gene fragments that are pieced together in order to generate an antibody gene. During the process the 'unwanted' DNA is spliced out and is lost forever. Therefore the DNA pattern using an immunoglobulin probe before the gene has rearranged is quite different to that generated after the gene has rearranged.

Southern blotting is also used in the diagnosis of globin gene disorders, and in particular sickle cell anaemia and thalassaemia. In sickle cell anaemia the mutation affects a single restriction site within the β-globin gene and the Southern blot pattern is quite characteristic for normal and mutated β-globin locus. Thalassaemia is much more complex but many mutations and deletions have been characterized using Southern blot hybridization. Many of these studies have been replaced by PCR analysis, which provides a faster result than Southern blotting, which may take several days.

Northern blotting

This is performed in a similar manner using RNA instead of DNA, i.e. RNA is size-separated on agarose gel, blotted onto filters and immobilized and finally probed using a radiolabelled gene probe. The location and size of the desired RNA species will be detected autoradiographically.

PCR amplification of DNA sequences

Southern blotting is a useful technique for assessing whether there is a clone of abnormal cells in blood, marrow or other tissue but is not useful if these cells are present in only very small amounts. In this case techniques that involve amplification of specific DNA sequences are required. PCR has filled the void in this respect and has found a place in diagnostic laboratories investigating oncogenes, haematological malignancies, general medicine, infectious disease, etc. In fact, PCR has been adopted by most medical specialties within a short period of time, considering that the technique has only been in common use for about 5 years. Part of the attraction of a PCR-based approach is its extreme simplicity and the speed with which results are obtained.

In essence, two short DNA primers on either side of the gene of interest bind to the fragment of interest (Figure 7.6). The region between the primers is filled in using a heat-stable DNA polymerase (Taq polymerase). After a single round of amplification has been performed the whole process is repeated. This takes place 30 times (i.e. through 30 cycles of amplification) and leads to (theoretically) a million-fold increase in the amount of specific sequence. After the 30 cycles are complete a sample of the PCR reaction is run on agarose gel. Information about the presence or absence of the region or mutation of interest is obtained by assessing the size and number of different PCR products obtained after 30 cycles of amplification.

PCR is currently used to amplify immunoglobulin genes, HIV loci, tuberculosis genes and many other targets that are of use in molecular medicine. PCR is a rapid diagnostic technique which does not rely on large quantities of starting DNA template. The quality of DNA need not be high and for this reason PCR amplification of genes is being performed more and

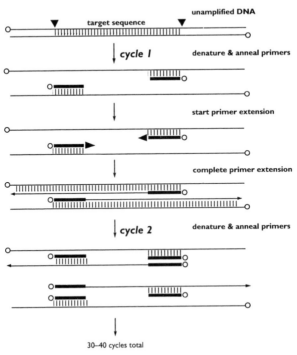

Fig. 7.6   PCR amplification of DNA

Examples of the use of PCR amplification in clinical medicine

Virology	Detection of EBV, HIV and other viruses
Bacteriology	Detection of bacterial pathogens, including mycobacteria
Histopathology	Oncogene mutations and gene expression
Haematology	T-cell receptor and immunoglobulin gene rearrangements, minimal residual disease detection, oncogene expression and mutation, globin gene analysis
General	Detection of novel mutations
	Detection of known mutations, e.g. Duchenne muscular dystrophy, cystic fibrosis, myotonic dystrophy, fragile X syndrome
	Detection of fetal blood groups and other genes using DNA extracted from amniocyte, e.g. rhesus, Kell and Duffy groups
	Detection of mutations predisposing to cancer and myocardial infarction
	HLA typing

more on archival pathology specimens. PCR can be used to quantitate mRNA species in blood samples and tissue samples. Unfortunately, to date no satisfactory DNA-based quantitative methods have been designed that are satisfactory for routine use.

Modifications of the PCR technique

ARMS PCR

This is the amplification refractory mutations system. In this form of PCR one of the oligonucleotide primers is designed so that its 3' terminal residue lies precisely at a point mutation site. PCR is carried out in duplicate: in one reaction the primers used match the normal sequence; in the other the primer matches the mutant sequence. By comparing the band(s) obtained in each reaction the presence or absence of a point mutation will be detected. ARMS PCR is used extensively in the analysis of β-globin gene mutations in β-thalassaemia (ARMS PCR is not useful in α-thalassaemia since these disorders are caused primarily by gene deletions rather than point mutations).

RACE PCR

This is rapid amplification of cDNA ends. The reaction uses one primer designed on the basis of a given protein sequence and a second primer which flanks the cloning site in a phage or plasmid vector. The substrate used is a total cDNA library (derived from cellular mRNA species). The technique is useful for identifying 5′ terminal cDNA sequences.

In situ hybridization *and* FISH

In situ hybridization grew out of standard cytogenetic analysis of metaphase chromosomes in which metaphase chromosomes were prepared on glass slides to which specific labelled probes were applied. The location of binding of the probe was detected by visualizing the signal produced after coating the slides with a photographic emulsion, which generated a black area around the probe which was labelled with ^{32}P. *In situ* hybridization has been further refined and has been applied to tissue sections and other materials using DNA probes for specific genes. *In situ* hybridization has also been adapted to work with mRNA in tissue samples.

FISH is a further modification based on the original principles, whereby specific gene probes are hybridized to chromosomes without the need for metaphase preparations; instead interphase cells may be used. This allows a far greater number of cells to be examined than could otherwise be done using metaphase chromosome preparations. Instead of ^{32}P the probes are labelled with fluorescent dye and hybridization may be detected as red or blue dots over the cells.

FISH has been used extensively in the analysis of trisomies and monosomies associated with specific leukaemias and lymphomas. The presence of trisomy is detected as three fluorescent dots within the cell whilst monosomy is seen as a single fluorescent dot within the cell. FISH has been used widely within paediatric leukaemias, such as ALL, where abnormalities of chromosome number are common.

Cloning and sequencing genes

DNA sequencing, previously a laborious and intensive process, is now automated and streamlined. DNA fragments such as those generated by polymerase chain amplification may be sequenced using automated DNA-sequencing equipment which uses fluorescent dyes, a different colour for each base, to produce computer-generated printouts that can be imported directly into DNA analysis software. This allows comparison of the sequence with published sequences and the detection of frameshift mutations, deletions, inversion and other abnormal rearrangement patterns. These fragments of DNA can often be sequenced directly without any prior manipulation. Occasionally cloning is required.

Cloning today is equally straightforward and several companies provide reagents and plasmids for cloning purposes. In these a plasmid of known DNA sequence is ligated to the sequence of interest and transfected into competent *Escherichia coli*. These bacteria are then grown on agar plates. The bacteria that have taken up the plasmid DNA containing the cloned fragment appear as white colonies on the agar (due to disruption of a gene during the cloning process; those bacteria with plasmid but no DNA sequence appear blue). The plasmid containing the cloned DNA is purified and sequenced using a similar method to that used for direct sequencing. Cloning is of value when a leukaemic or other malignant sequence is being sought in a blood or marrow sample. If 10 bacterial colonies are analysed and three contain an identical cloned sequence for, e.g. immunoglobulin genes, then this sequence must represent that of the leukaemic cell population – it is highly unlikely that three cells would each rearrange their immunoglobulin genes in exactly the same way, since there are large numbers of germline variable, diversity, joining and constant region genes to select when these genes are undergoing somatic recombination.

Cloning genes and analysis of their sequences has proved of great interest and value commercially (see page 270). The fine structure of introns, exons, leader sequences and promoter regions has been elucidated through painstaking cloning of gene libraries and assembling entire genes from cloned fragments. Some cloned genes have been introduced into artificial systems (e.g. Chinese hamster ovary or bacterial systems) to produce large quantities of protein for human use. These proteins include insulin, erythropoietin, many other hormones, recombinant clotting proteins and many enzymes.

The future of molecular biology within medicine

The next few years will see many improvements of existing techniques. Automation will become more common; commercial products arising out of molecular biological research will become cheaper and the range more extensive than ever before.

Examples of pharmaceutical products obtained by expression cloning

Gene product	Disease treated
FVIII	Haemophilia A
FIX	Haemophilia B
Factor VIIa	Inhibitors in haemophilia A and B
Erythropoietin	Anaemia, e.g. in chronic renal failure
Insulin	Diabetes mellitus
Growth hormone	Growth hormone deficiency
Tissue plasminogen activator	Thrombosis
Hepatitis B vaccine	Hepatitis B
Interferon-α	CML, HCL, chronic hepatitis
Interferon-β	MS
Interferon-γ	Infections in patients with chronic granulomatous disease
G/GM-CSF	Neutropenia
DNAse	Cystic fibrosis

Biology and utility of recombinant clotting factors

Haemophilia A (FVIII deficiency) affects around 1 in 5000 males; haemophilia B (FIX deficiency) affects 1 in 25 000 males. Both diseases are associated with spontaneous bleeding into joints and muscles. People who are mildly affected may only bleed when they undergo bleeding associated with trauma, e.g. surgery. In both disorders there is no single genotype and the deficiencies may be caused by partial gene deletions, point mutations causing nonsense mutations or premature stop codons in the gene. In most patients the genetic defect is not known.

In 1964 it was discovered that FVIII was present in cryoprecipitate and this allowed treatment of haemophilia A for the first time. Subsequently, FVIII was purified and ultimately lyophilized and highly purified FVIII became available. The concentrates, however, are made from large pools of plasma involving many different donors. By the 1970s reports of viral infection appeared. The major agents transmitted by purified coagulation factors are hepatitis B and C, as well as HIV. The risk of infection is reduced by heavily screening donors and immunizing haemophiliacs against hepatitis B. There have also been great improvements in the methods involved in the purification and sterilization of factor concentrates but the infection risk is still present. There has therefore been great interest in the use of molecular biological approaches in producing factor concentrates for human use.

FVIII

This is a glycoprotein that circulates in plasma non-covalently bound to von Willebrand factor. Activated FVIII plays a key role in the intrinsic coagulation pathway as a cofactor for FIXa. FVIII has been investigated following the successful cloning of the gene.

FVIII comprises multiple polypeptides of 80–120 kDa. The 80 kDa fraction comprises the C terminal of the light chain and a 92–210 kDa fraction is derived from the N-terminal region. The gene for FVIII has been characterized and is 186 000 bp in size with 26 exons (from 69 to 3106 bp) and 25 introns (207–32,4000 bp). The mRNA for FVIII is 9 kb in size. The cDNA derived from the mRNA encodes 2351 amino acids. The cDNA has been expressed in two mammalian systems: baby hamster kidney (by Genentech) and Chinese hamster ovary (by Genetics Institute). These mammalian systems have allowed the study of FVIII synthesis, processing and secretion.

The molecule is synthesized as a single 2351 amino acid chain, from which a 19 amino acid signal polypeptide is cleaved. The 2332 amino acid protein is arranged into three domains: 3 × A domains, 1 × B domain and 2 × C domains. The mature protein shares 40% homology with factor V and caeruloplasmin.

During transit through the endoplasmic reticulum high mannose sugars are added to multiple asparagine residues (especially in the B domain). von Willebrand factor is required for survival of FVIII. In cell culture systems the presence of serum containing von Willebrand factor is needed for accumulation of FVIII. A comparison of recombinant FVIII and plasma-derived FVIII has shown that they are identical molecules.

Recombinant FVIII is secreted as 200 and 80 kDa chains which require von Willebrand factor for their association. The recombinant FVIII has identical peptides generated by thrombin/factor Xa and activated protein C to the native protein. Recombinant FVIII has an identical glycosylation pattern to native FVIII and the rFVIII corrects the clotting time of haemophilic plasma. Similarly the activity of recombinant FVIII is increased by thrombin and activity is reduced by activated protein C, and by anti-FVIII antibodies. Recombinant FVIII binds reversibly to immobilized von Willebrand factor.

Recombinant FVIII secreted into culture medium is purified by ion exchange chromatography and immunoaffinity chromatography. The final product is lyophilized and stabilized using human albumin. The product contains trace amounts of mammalian proteins (mouse and hamster).

FIX

This is a serine protease and is defective or reduced in haemophilia B. FIX is converted to FIXa by the intrinsic pathway or by tissue factor. The molecule is a 415 amino acid glycoprotein and is synthesized in the liver as a 461 amino acid precursor with a 29 amino acid signal peptide.

FIX requires several post-translational modification steps for full functional activity, e.g. vitamin K-dependent carboxylation of the 12 N-terminal glutamic acid residues to carboxyglutamyl residues required for calcium binding.

The gene for FIX and a cDNA copy were cloned successfully in 1982. The sequence was fully described in 1985. The gene is 33 kb long with 8 exons and 7 introns.

A recombinant FIX molecule has been developed by Genetics Institute and is currently undergoing clinical trials in the USA and Europe.

Recombinant factor VIIa

This product has a role in the management of patients with haemophilia who have antibodies to infused FVIII or FIX. This is seen in 10–20% of patients with haemophilia A and 1% of patients with haemophilia B. This makes treatment of bleeding episodes difficult, especially if the antibody is high titre. To date, various strategies have been used, e.g. porcine FVIII, FVIII inhibitor bypassing, immune tolerance induction using continuous treatment with FVIII and immunosuppression. Factor VII has been used to treat bleeds in patients with FVIII deficiency and more recently recombinant factor VII has been synthesized. A cDNA coding for factor VII was characterized in 1986 following screening of cDNA libraries.

The recombinant protein is purified and during the process the factor VII is activated to generate recombinant FVIIa. There are minor differences between recombinant FVIIa and the native protein, most particularly in the glycosylation and γ-carboxylation. Preclinical trials were successful and the product is now available for clinical use in haemophilia A and B with inhibitors. The product does not require stabilization with albumin and is entirely blood-free. Unfortunately, the half-life is very short and i.v. injections need to be given every 2–3 h in order to control bleeding.

The future

Genetic research and manipulation may enable modification of the natural structure of coagulation molecules, e.g. to increase the half-life by manufacturing molecules resistant to proteolysis. Trials involving a modified FVIII with deleted B domain are currently in progress. Hybrid coagulation proteins (e.g. human and porcine) are being developed and these may generate molecules with increased resistance to circulating inhibitors.

References

Dameshek, W., Rubio, F., Mahoney, J. et al. (1958) Treatment of idiopathic thrombocytopenic purpura (ITP). JAMA, 166: 1805–15.

Dahlback, B. (1995) Factor V gene mutation causing inherited resistance to activated protein C as a basis for venous thromboembolism. Journal of Internal Medicine, 237: 221–7.

8 Examination lists

Leukaemia and lymphoma

Classification of cytotoxic agents and mode of action

Class of drug	Mode of action
Alkylating agents	
Cyclophosphamide	Cross-link double-stranded DNA
Chlorambucil	Prevent RNA production
Busulphan	
Melphalan	
Corticosteroids	
	Modify gene expression
	↓ Prostaglandin and leukotriene production
	Membrane damage
Interferons	
Interferon-α	Induce 2, 5-oligoA synthetase
Interferon-γ	polymerize ATP residues into short oligomers leading to mRNA degradation
	Activate RNA breakdown
Antimetabolites	
Methotrexate	Inhibits dihydrofolate reductase
6 Mercaptopurine	Inhibits purine synthesis
6 Thioguanine	Incorporates into DNA → strand breaks
Hydroxyurea	Inhibits ribonucleotide reductase
5-Azacytidine	Inhibits pyrimidine synthesis
Vinca alkaloids	
Vincristine	Bind tubulin
Vindesine	Inhibit microtubule polymerization
Vinblastine	which is needed for spindle formation

Anthracyclines

Daunorubicin	Inhibits topoisomerase II
Hydroxydaunorubicin (Adriamycin)	Free radical generators
Mitozantrone	DNA intercalators
M-amsacrine	

Enzyme inhibitors

2-Deoxycoformycin	Purine analogue
	Inhibits adenosine deaminase
	dATP accumulates
	NAD is depleted
2-CDA	Purine analogue
	Causes death by apoptosis
Fludarabine	Purine analogue
	Inhibits adenosine deaminase
L-asparaginase	Hydrolyses L-asparagine and inhibits protein synthesis
VP16 (etoposide)	Inhibits topo II and induces double-stranded DNA breaks

Disorders predisposing to acute leukaemia

Disorder	Leukaemia
Myeloproliferative disease	AML predominantly
Myelodysplasia	AML
HTLV-1 infection	Acute T cell leukaemia/lymphoma
Down's syndrome	ALL or AML
Fanconi's anaemia	AML
Ataxia telangiectasia	ALL, NHL
Aplastic anaemia	ALL mainly, AML
PNH	AML mainly
Chemotherapy/radiotherapy	MDS → AML

AML FAB subtypes

M0	Undifferentiated, negative cytochemistry, identified by McAbs and electron microscopy
M1	Myeloblastic, no maturation
M2	Myeloblastic with maturation
M2 baso	M2 with basophil blasts
M3	Hypergranular promyelocytic
M3 variant	Hypogranular promyelocytic
M4	Acute myelomonocytic (granulocyte and monocyte differentiation)
M4 eo	M4 with marrow eosinophilia
M5	Acute monocytic
M6	Erythroleukaemia
M7	Acute megakaryoblastic leukaemia

MDS FAB Subtype	Marrow blasts (%)
RA	<5
RARS	<5
RAEB	5–20
RAEB-t	20–30
CMML	<20

>30% marrow blasts indicates progression to AML

Prognostic Factors in ALL

	Bad	Good
WBC	>50 × 10^9/l	<10 × 10^9/l
Age	<2 years, ≥15 years	2–10 years
Sex	Male	Female
Karyotype	t(8;14) = L3 subtype t(4;11) = null ALL t(9;22) hypodiploid	>50 chromosomes, i.e. hyperdipoloid
Morphology	L2 and L3 subtypes	L1
Cell markers	B cell (SmIg$^+$)	common ALL
Others	CNS leukaemia Organomegaly	Remission within 4 weeks of therapy

Cell markers in the classification of ALL

Marker	null	cALL	pre-B	B-ALL	pre-T	T-ALL
CD2	−	−	−	−	−	+
CD3	−	−	−	−	+	+
CD7	−	−	−	−	+	+
CD10	−	+	+	−/+	−/+	−
CD19	+	+	+	+	−	−
CD22	+	+	+	+	−	−
Cyto μ	−	−	+	+	−	−
SmIg	−	−	−	+	−	−
HLA DR	+	+	+	+	−/+	−
TdT	+	+	+	−/+	+	+
CD34	+	+	+	−	−	−

Cell markers in the classification of AML

Marker	M0	M1	M2/3	M4/5	M6	M7
CD34	+	+	+/−	+/−	−	+
CD13	+	+	+	+	+	+
CD33	+	+	+	+	+	+
CD11b	−	−	+	+	−	−
CD14	−	−	−	+	−	−
Glycophorin	−	−	−	−	+	−
TdT	−/+	−/+	−	−	−	−

Cell markers in the classification of chronic B cell leukaemia and NHL

Marker	CLL	PLL	HCL	SLVL	FL	PCL
Surface Ig	+	++	++	++	++	−
Cyto Ig	−	−/+	−/++	−/++	−	++
CD5	+	−/+	−	−	−	−
CD22	−/+	++	++	++	++	−
CD19	++	++	++	++	++	−
CD10	−	−/+	−	−	+	−/+
CD38	−	−	−	−	−	+

Cell markers in the classification of mature T cell leukaemias

Marker	T-CLL	T-PLL	ATLL	Sézary
CD2	+	+	+	−
CD3	+	+/−	+	+
CD4	−	+/−	+	+
CD8	+	−/+	−	−
CD5	−	+	+	+
CD7	−/+	++	−	−
CD25	−	−/+	++	−/+

Salmon-Durie staging criteria for multiple myeloma

Major	Minor
Plasmacytoma on biopsy	Marrow with >10< 30% plasma cells
Marrow with >30% plasma cells	Monoclonal spike but less than level defined for major
Monoclonal globulin spike:	Lytic bone lesions
>35 g/l for IgG	Normal serum:
>20 g/l for IgA	IgM <0.5 g/l
>1 g/24 h Bence Jones proteinuria	IgA <1.0 g/l
	IgG <6.0 g/l

Definition of equivocal myelomatosis

1. There are minimal/no symptoms attributable to myelomatosis.
2. The pre-transfusion Hb is >10 g/dl.
3. The post-rehydration serum creatinine is <130 μmol/l.
4. There are no osteolytic lesions other than minimal lesions which do not threaten pathological fracture and are not associated with pain.
5. Plasma cells comprise <25% of the mononuclear cells in the marrow which shows normal haematopoietic activity.
6. Serum β_2-microglobulin is <4 mg/l.
7. There is <1 g of free light chain excretion per gram of creatinine.
8. There are no objective factors which indicate that the patient has progressive myelomatosis.

Miscellaneous

Causes of elevated platelet count (>450 × 10⁹/l)	Causes of reduced platelet count (<150 × 10⁹/l)
Essential thrombocythaemia	Myelodysplasia
Chronic granulocytic leukaemia	Alloimmune thrombocytopenia in
Myelofibrosis (early)	infancy
Polycythaemia rubra vera	Isoimmune thrombocytopenia in infancy
Myelodysplasia (especially 5q⁻	ITP
syndrome)	Post-infection (especially viral)
Infection	HIV infection
Inflammation	PTP
Active bleeding	DIC
Trauma	Autoimmune
Postoperative	Drug-induced
Early post-splenectomy	Alcohol-induced
Iron deficiency	Hypersplenism

Factors increasing iron absorption	Factors decreasing iron absorption
Acid	Alkali
Inorganic iron	Organic iron
Fe^{2+}	Fe^{3+}
Iron deficiency	Agents precipitating iron, e.g. phytates
Pregnancy	Excess iron
Adolescence	Infections
Bleeding	Inflammatory disorders
Primary haemochromatosis	Gastrectomy/achlorhydria

Schilling test interpretation

	Excretion of labelled vitamin B_{12}	
	Part I	Part II
Normal	>8%	
Vegan	>8%	>8%
Pernicious anaemia	<8%	>8%
Blind loops	<8%	No change
Malabsorption	<8%	No change

Causes of intravascular haemolysis	Causes of extravascular haemolysis
Traumatic haemolysis	Autoimmune haemolytic anaemias
Type A– G6PD deficiency	Hereditary spherocytosis
Haemolytic transfusion reaction	Liver disease
e.g. ABO Incompatibility	Pyruvate kinase deficiency
PNH	Unstable haemoglobins
Infection, e.g. *Plasmodium*	

Polycythaemia

Polycythaemia rubra vera
High altitude
Cigarette smoking
Chronic obstructive airways disease
Cyanotic heart disease
Sleep apnoea syndromes
High-affinity haemoglobins
Renal carcinoma
Uterine fibroids
Cerebellar haemangioblastoma
Familial
Apparent

Causes of splenomegaly

Neoplastic disease	Lymphoma
	Leukaemia (CML, CLL, HCL)
	Myelofibrosis
	PRV
	Metastatic disease
Infection	Viral (infectious mononucleosis, hepatitis)
	Bacterial (tuberculosis, brucellosis, syphilis)
	Fungal (histoplasmosis)
	Parasitic (toxoplasmosis, malaria, schistosomiasis, *Echinococcus*)
	Rickettsial (Rocky Mountain spotted fever)
Infiltration	Sarcoidosis
	Amyloidosis
Inflammation	Rheumatoid (Felty's syndrome)
	Sarcoidosis
	SLE

Haemolytic diseases	Thalassaemia
	HbC
	Hereditary spherocytosis and elliptocytosis
	Immune haemolytic anaemias
Miscellaneous	Gaucher's disease
	Niemann–Pick disease
	Severe iron-deficiency anaemia
	Idiopathic

Hyposplenism

With atrophic spleen	Coeliac disease/dermatitis herpetiformis
	Ulcerative colitis
	Crohn's disease
	GVHD
	Sickle cell anaemia (post-infancy)
With normal/large spleen	Sarcoidosis
	Amyloidosis
Miscellaneous	Post-splenectomy

Low-molecular-weight versus standard heparin

Low-molecular-weight heparin	Standard heparin
Average molecular weight <10 kDa	Glycosaminoglycan mixture
Does not prolong APTT	Molecular weight 15 kDa
Measure activity by anti-Xa assay	Prolongs APTT
Higher anti-Xa than antithrombin effect	Use APTT to monitor
Longer half-life (> 30 min)	Binds antithrombin III
↓ Tissue plasminogen activator activity	Inactivates Xa
Greater bioavailability than standard	Half-life 30 min
Too small to inactivate IIa well	
More difficult to reverse with protamine	
Monitoring: Xa assay most useful	
Once-daily dosage	

Antithrombin III deficiency

Hereditary
Oestrogens
Pregnancy
Liver disease
Nephrotic syndrome
DIC
Heparin therapy

Factors absent from aged normal serum and adsorbed plasma

Normal	Aged serum	Adsorbed plasma
I	~~I~~	I
II	~~II~~	~~II~~
V	~~V~~	V
VII	VII	~~VII~~
VIII	~~VIII~~	VIII
IX	IX	~~IX~~
X	X	~~X~~
XI	XI	XI
XII	XII	XII

Roman numerals with strikethrough (e.g. ~~II~~) indicate that this factor is missing in this type of control plasma or serum. Aged serum lacks the labile coagulation proteins whilst adsorbed plasma consists of plasma from which the vitamin K-dependent factors (II, VII, IX and X) have been adsorbed onto aluminium hydroxide. Adding these reagents to plasma samples of patients with suspected factor deficiencies (i.e. with prolonged PT or APTT) in PT or APTT assays allows one to form a 'best guess' regarding the deficient factor, depending on whether or not the aged serum or adsorbed plasma corrects the deficiency.

↑ Warfarin effect	↓ Warfarin effect
Alcohol	Barbiturates
Antibiotics	Phenytoin
NSAIDs	Spironolactone
Aspirin	Griseofulvin
Tolbutamide	Oral contraceptive
Antidepressants	
Allopurinol	
Laxatives	
Quinine	
Thyroxine	

Causes of vitamin B_{12} deficiency	Causes of folate deficiency
Pernicious anaemia	Dietary, elderly, alcoholic
Nutritional, vegans	Malabsorption, coeliac, Crohn's disease
Stagnant loops	Anticonvulsant therapy
Ileal resection	Pregnancy
Crohn's disease	Haemolysis
Gastrectomy	Liver disease
Coeliac disease	
Fish tapeworm	

↑ Serum ferritin	↓ Serum ferritin
Idiopathic haemochromatosis	Iron deficiency
Iron-loading anaemia, e.g. thalassaemia	Pregnancy
Multiple transfusion	Hypothyroid
Megaloblastic anaemia	Ascorbate deficiency
Hypoplastic anaemia	
Inflammation	
Infection	
Hepatoma	
Neoplasia	

Spherocytosis – causes

Hereditary spherocytosis
Warm autoimmune haemolytic anaemia
Delayed transfusion reaction
Immediate transfusion reaction
ABO HDN
Rhesus HDN
Burns
Drug-induced haemolytic anaemia
Zieve's syndrome
Post-splenectomy/hyposplenism
Microangiopathic haemolytic anaemia
Heinz body anaemias

Causes of ↑ HbF

β-Thalassaemia
Sickle cell anaemia
Hb Lepore
Fanconi's anaemia
Juvenile CML
AML in children

Causes of elevated HbA_2 ($\alpha_2\delta_2$)	Causes of reduced HbA_2 ($\alpha_2\delta_2$)
β-Thalassaemia trait	δβ-Thalassaemia (Lepore)
β-Thalassaemia major	HbH disease (β_4)
Megaloblastic anaemia	Severe iron-deficiency anaemia
Unstable Hb	Sideroblastic anaemia (some cases)
	Hereditary persistence of HbF

Methaemoglobinaemia

Congenital causes	Acquired causes
Newborn (sensitive to oxidizing agents) NADH metHb reductase deficiency M haemoglobins, e.g. abnormal α chains	Oxidants (amyl nitrate, chlorate) Chronic intravascular haemolysis

Haemoglobin production during development

Embryo

Hb Gower 1 $(\zeta_2\varepsilon_2)$ Hb Gower 2 $(\alpha_2\varepsilon_2)$ Hb Portland $(\zeta_2\gamma_2)$	from 0 to 10 weeks

Fetus

HbF $(\alpha_2\gamma_2)$	85%
HbA $(\alpha_2\beta_2)$	5–10%

Adult

HbA $(\alpha_2\beta_2)$	97%
HbA2 $(\alpha_2\delta_2)$	2.5%
HbF $(\alpha_2\gamma_2)$	0.5%

Lymphocyte disorders

T cell	B cell
Di George's syndrome (absent T cells) Wiskott–Aldrich Chédiak–Higashi	Ataxia telangiectasia Chédiak–Higashi Chronic granulomatous disease

Pure red cell aplasia

Congenital	Acquired
Diamond–Blackfan syndrome Reduced Hb and reticulocytes at birth Marrow shows no erythroid precursors BFU-E reduced or absent Treatment – steroids, blood transfusion	Idiopathic Autoimmune, e.g. SLE Thymoma (in 30–50% patients) T cell lymphocytosis CLL Lymphoma Drugs

Sideroblastic anaemia

Congenital
Acquired
   Primary acquired (myelodysplasia)
   Secondary acquired:
      B_6 deficiency (coeliac, pregnancy)
      B_6 antagonists (isoniazid)
      Lead poisoning
      Chloramphenicol
      Alcoholism

Disorders associated with marrow fibrosis

Myelofibrosis
Infections, e.g. tuberculosis, osteomyelitis
Lymphomas
Occasionally CGL
Metastatic carcinoma (prostate, breast)
Acute leukaemia (some)
Irradiation
Benzene, fluorine, lead
Paget's disease
Osteopetrosis

Erythropoietin side-effects
(in patients with renal failure particularly)

Elevated BP
Fits
Thrombosis at vascular access site
Myalgia
Skin irritation
Iron deficiency
Headache
Nausea/vomiting
Breathlessness
Diarrhoea
Abdominal and loin pain

Morphological abnormalities and variants

Dimorphic film	Iron deficiency responding to iron Patients with mixed deficiency Sideroblastic anaemia Post-transfusion Post-splenectomy
Polychromatic red cells	Response to blood loss Response to haematinic treatment Haemolysis Marrow infiltration
Microcytes	Iron deficiency Thalassaemia major Thalassaemia minor Sickle cell trait $\delta\beta$-Thalassaemia HbH disease HbC trait HbSC disease HbE trait Sideroblastic anaemia Anaemia of chronic disorders
Macrocytes	Vitamin B_{12} or folate deficiency Reticulocytosis Hypothyroidism Liver disease Alcoholism Myeloma Cytotoxic drugs Leukoerythroblastic anaemia Sideroblastic anaemia Aplastic anaemia Myelodysplasia Chronic respiratory failure Pregnancy Newborn
Spherocytes	Warm antibody autoimmune haemolytic anaemia Hereditary spherocytosis Delayed transfusion reaction ABO HDN Burns Zieve's syndrome Post-splenectomy

Elliptocytes	Hereditary elliptocytosis Myeloproliferative disease Myelodysplasia
Pencil cells	Iron-deficiency anaemia Thalassaemia Megaloblastic anaemia Myelofibrosis Pyruvate kinase deficiency
Fragmented red cells	Microangiopathic haemolytic anaemia DIC
Crenated red cells	Post-splenectomy
Teardrop red cells (poikilocytes)	Myelofibrosis Marrow infiltration (e.g. carcinoma) Thalassaemia Myelodysplasia Megaloblastic anaemia
Burr cells	Renal failure
Acanthocytes	Hereditary acanthocytosis a-β-lipoproteinaemia McLeod red cell phenotype Chronic liver disease (especially Zieve's syndrome)
Basophilic stippling	Megaloblastic anaemia Lead poisoning MDS Haemoglobinopathies
Rouleaux	Cold agglutinins Chronic inflammation Paraproteinaemia Myeloma
Increased reticulocytes	Bleeding Haemolysis Marrow infiltration Sudden severe hypoxia
Heinz bodies	Composed of denatured Hb Stain with methyl violet or new methylene blue Not seen in normals (removed by spleen) Small numbers seen post-splenectomy Seen with oxidant drugs G6PD deficiency Sulphonamides Unstable haemoglobins (Hb Zurich, Köln)

Howell–Jolly bodies	Composed of DNA
	Generally removed by the spleen
	Dyserythropoietic states, e.g. B_{12} deficiency, myelodysplasia
	Post-splenectomy

H bodies	= HbH inclusions
	Composed of denatured HbH (β_4 tetramer)
	Stain with methylene blue
	Seen in HbH disease ($--/-\alpha$)
	Less prominent in α-thalassaemia trait
	Not present in normal subjects

Pappenheimer bodies	Iron granules in red cells
	Detect using Perls' stain (potassium ferrocyanide)

Hyposplenic blood film	Howell–Jolly bodies
	Target cells
	Occasional nucleated red blood cells
	Lymphocytosis
	Macrocytosis
	Acanthocytes
	Pappenheimer bodies (containing iron)
	Occasional spherocytes

Atypical lymphocytes	Infectious mononucleosis
	Acute leukaemia
	ALL
	Hepatitis
	Measles
	Tuberculosis
	Toxoplasmosis
	Drug reactions

Auer rods	AML (M2 and M3 usually)

Chédiak–Higashi	Autosomal recessive
	Large grey inclusions in WBC and other body cells
	Anaemia, neutropenia, thrombocytopenia

Alder–Reilly	Autosomal recessive
	Dark purple inclusions in WBC

Döhle bodies	Small blue cytoplasmic inclusions in neutrophils
	Found in:
	May–Hegglin anomaly
	Familial
	Pregnancy
	Infection
	Burns
	MDS
	AML

Leukoerythroblastic film	Metastatic infiltration of bone marrow: Breast Prostate Lung Thyroid Renal Acute leukaemia Lymphoma Myelofibrosis Myeloma Acute haemolysis HDN Sickle crisis
May–Hegglin anomaly	Basophilic cytoplasmic inclusions in WBC Autosomal dominant
Pelger–Huët neutrophil	Neutrophils with bilobed nuclei Familial Autosomal dominant Acquired abnormality in MDS
Sickle cells	Sickle cell disease HbSC disease
Target cells	Obstructive jaundice Liver disease HbC trait and disease HbE trait and disease HbD trait and disease HbH disease Sickle cell anaemia HbSC disease β-Thalassaemia trait and major Iron-deficiency anaemia Hereditary persistence of HbF
Bite cells	Oxidant drugs Haemolysis in G6PD deficiency HbC disease

Blood changes in pregnancy

Hb, PCV and RCC ↓ due to ↑ plasma volume
Lowest levels by 30 weeks' gestation
Hb generally ≥10 g/dl unless there is another underlying problem
or deficiency

↑ Eosinophils in peripheral blood

Atopic individuals, including eczema, asthma, allergic rhinitis
Aspergillosis
Other fungal infections
Pemphigus/pemphigoid
Drug hypersensitivity
Parasitic infestations: schistosomiasis, filariasis, cysticercosis, trichinosis, larva migrans, etc.
Hodgkin's disease
Chronic granulocytic leukaemia
Carcinoma

↑ Basophils in peripheral blood

Chronic granulocytic leukaemia
PRV
Myelofibrosis
ET
Hypothyroidism
Ulcerative colitis
Oestrogens

↑ Monocytes in peripheral blood

Chronic infections, e.g. tuberculosis
Chronic inflammation, e.g. Crohn's disease, ulcerative colitis, rheumatoid, SLE
Carcinomas
Myeloproliferative diseases
MDS
CMML
CML
Juvenile CML
Long-term haemodialysis

Blood transfusion

Uses of IVIg

Childhood ITP
Adult ITP response is usually good but not sustained
ITP of pregnancy
Neonatal alloimmune and isoimmune thrombocytopenia (NAIT)
Post-transfusion purpura (PTP)
Secondary immune thrombocytopenia (SLE, HIV)
Autoimmune haemolytic anaemia
Autoimmune thrombocytopenia
Autoimmune neutropenia
Acquired clotting disorders
Primary hypogammaglobulinaemia
Secondary immunodeficiency (CLL, myeloma)
Prophylaxis against bacterial infection in children with HIV
Parvovirus-induced aplasia
Coagulation factor autoantibody
Maternal antenatal treatment of RhD haemolytic disease

Complications of IVIg administration

Fever, chills, occasionally more severe constitutional symptoms
Commoner in hypogammaglobulinaemic patients when infected
Severe reactions due to IgA deficiency
Reactions can induce miscarriage
Haemolysis with transient positive DAT
Thrombotic episodes in elderly patients with ITP

Rhesus genotypes and incidence

Weiner notation		Fisher–Race notation
R_1R_1		CDe/CDe
R_2R_2		cDE/cDE
R_1r		CDe/cde
R_2r		cDE/cde
rr		cde/cde
r'r		Cde/cde
r"r		cdE/cde
R means	D	
r means	d	
1 or ' means	C	
2 or " means	E	

Haplotype		Frequency in population
R_1	CDe	Common
R_2	cDE	Common
R_z	CDE	Rare
R_o	cDe	2%
r'	Cde	1%
r"	cdE	1%
r_y	CdE	Very rare
r	cde	Common

Red cell antigen expression at birth

Weak	Normal
I	Rhesus
$Le^a Le^b$	Kell
A	Duffy (Fy)
B	Jk
P_1	MNSs
$Lu^a Lu^b$	

Protein blood groups	Carbohydrate blood groups
Rhesus	ABO
Kell	P
Duffy	Lewis
Kidd	Ii
MNSs	
Lutheran	

Fresh frozen plasma

Definite indications:

Single factor replacement if no specific concentrate available
Warfarin reversal
DIC
Thrombotic thrombocytopenic purpura

Conditional use*

Massive transfusion
Liver disease
Cardiopulmonary bypass
Special paediatric indications

* in presence of bleeding/disturbed coagulation

No justification for use

Hypovolaemia
Plasma exchange
'Formula' replacement
Nutritional support
Treatment of immunodeficiency

Apheresis

Indications for plasmapheresis

Hyperviscosity syndrome
Myasthenia gravis
Goodpasture's syndrome
Acute Guillain–Barré syndrome
Cryoglobulinaemia
Thrombotic thrombocytopenic purpura
Haemophilia with inhibitors
Refsum's disease
Cold agglutinin haemolytic anaemia
Some cases of poisoning

Occasionally useful

Familial hypercholesterolaemia
Immune complex vasculitis
Rapidly progressive glomerulonephritis
Rhesus haemolytic disease
Post-transfusion purpura
Bullous pemphigoid

Normal ranges for haematology, biochemistry and immunology

Haematology

Hb	13.0–18.0 g/dl (male)
	11.5–16.5 g/dl (female)
Haematocrit	0.40–0.52 (male)
	0.36–0.47 (female)
RCC	$4.5–6.5 \times 10^{12}/l$ (male)
	$3.8–5.8 \times 10^{12}/l$ (female)
MCV	77–95 fl
MCH	27.0–32.0 pg
MCHC	32.0–36.0 g/dl
WBC	$4.0–11.0 \times 10^9/l$
Neutrophils	$2.0–7.5 \times 10^9/l$
Lymphocytes	$1.5–4.5 \times 10^9/l$
Eosinophils	$0.04–0.4 \times 10^9/l$
Basophils	$0.0–0.1 \times 10^9/l$
Monocytes	$0.2–0.8 \times 10^9/l$
Platelets	$150–400 \times 10^9/l$
Reticulocytes	0.5–2.5% (or $50–100 \times 10^9/l$)
ESR	2–12 mm/1st hour (Westergren)
Serum B_{12}	150–700 ng/l
Serum folate	2.0–11.0 μg/l
Red cell folate	150–700 μg/l
Serum ferritin	15–300 μg/l (varies with sex and age)
	14–200 μg/l premenopausal female
INR	0.8–1.2
PT	12.0–14.0 s
APTR	0.8–1.2
APTT	26.0–33.5 s
Fibrinogen	2.0–4.0 g/l
Thrombin time	± 3 s of control
XDPs	<250 μg/l
Factors II, V, VII, VIII, IX, X, XI, XII	50–150 i.u./dl
RiCoF	45–150 i.u./dl
vWF: Ag	50–150 i.u./dl
Protein C	80–135 u/dl
Protein S	80–135 u/dl
Antithrombin III	80–120 u/dl
Bleeding time	3–9 min

Biochemistry

Serum urea	3.0–6.5 mmol/l
Serum creatinine	60–125 μmol/l
Serum sodium	135–145 mmol/l
Serum potassium	3.5–5.0 mmol/l
Serum albumin	32–50 g/l
Serum bilirubin	<17 μmol/l
Serum alkaline phosphatase	100–300 i.u./l
Serum calcium	2.15–2.55 mmol/l
Serum LDH	200–450 i.u./l
Serum phosphate	0.7–1.5 mmol/l
Serum total protein	63–80 g/l
Serum gamma glutamyl transferase	10–46 i.u./l
Serum iron	Male 14–33 μmol/l
	Female 11–28 μmol/l
Serum TIBC	45–75 μmol/l
Serum alanine aminotransferase	
Serum aspartate transaminase	5–42 i.u./l
Serum free T_4 (thyroxine)	9–24 pmol/l
Serum TSH	0.35–5.5 mU/l

Immunology

Immunoglobulins

IgG	5.3–16.5 g/l	
IgA	0.8–4.0 g/l	
IgM	0.5–2.0 g/l	
Complement	C3	0.89–2.09 g/l
	C4	0.12–0.53 g/l
	C_1 esterase	0.11–0.36 g/l
	CH_{50}	80–120%
C-reactive protein	<6 mg/l	
β_2-Microglobulin	serum	1.2–2.4 mg/l
CSF proteins	IgG	0.013–0.035 g/l
	Albumin	0.170–0.238 g/l
Urine proteins	Total protein	<150 mg/24 h
	Albumin (24-h)	<20 mg/24 h

Further Reading

MRCP

Hoffbrand, AV and Pettit, JE (1993) *Essential Haematology*, 3rd edn. Oxford: Blackwell Scientific Publications.

This is probably the best haematology text for the MRCP examination. The book is aimed at senior undergraduates and those with a general interest in haematology. The writing is crystal clear and the diagrams are beautifully drawn and illustrate the book well.

Hughes-Jones, NC and Wickramsinghe, SN (1996) *Lecture Notes on Haematology*, 6th edn. Oxford: Blackwell Science.

In previous editions this book was fairly uninspiring and was no competition for the others. However, in this, its sixth edition, the book has been completely overhauled and is a very readable account of the subject. It is compact and pitched for senior students/MRCP. We would recommend this book quite strongly for those wishing to get up to speed in haematology fairly quickly without being burdened by extraneous detail.

Bain, B (1996) *Blood Cells*. Oxford: Blackwell Science.

The first edition of this book was excellent but its weakness was the index, which had an excessive number of entries. The book has been rewritten and is now more functional, with a slimmed-down index. Sadly, some of the information present in the first book that made it so unusual (e.g. the examples of FBCs sprinkled throughout the text) is missing from the new edition. None the less, this book has sufficient high-quality photomicrographs to make it an excellent bench book and should be used in conjunction with the Hoffbrand atlas whenever morphological aspects of blood cells are being evaluated. The book also has an excellent section on the characteristics of the major automated blood counters.

Medicine International

This series is useful for MRCP Part 1 and 2. The haematology component is worth reading through and, although not exhaustive, does cover the major areas of malignant and non-malignant haematology.

MRCPath

Major texts

Beutler, E, Lichtman, MA, Coller, BS and Kipps, TJ (eds) (1995). *Williams Hematology*, 5th edn. New York: McGraw-Hill.

This is probably the best large haematology text available and has been extensively rewritten for the fifth edition. It is a useful reference source but may be read selectively for those aiming at the MRCPath written section.

Hoffbrand, AV & Lewis, SM (1989) *Postgraduate Haematology*, 3rd edn., Oxford: Heinemann.

This is the best British text in haematology but this edition is now somewhat outdated and a new edition is due in 1998. The chapters are written by leading authorities and are probably sufficient for MRCPath, although larger texts such as *Williams* will need to supplement those areas that are weak.

Hoffbrand, AV. and Pettit, JE (1994) *Sandoz Atlas, Clinical Haematology*, 2nd edn. London: Mosby-Wolfe.

Essential reading, as well as being the best atlas of haematological disease available. The quality of the photomicrographs and line drawings is unsurpassed by any other book to date.

Spivak, JL *et al.* (eds) *Yearbook of Hematology 1995*, St Louis: Mosby.

Published each year by Mosby, this (expensive at £58) volume summarizes the most relevant papers in haematology over the previous year. Authors, titles, source and abstract are provided. The main advantage of this book is that the authors have written a critique of almost every paper, which makes this a useful resource for vivas and essay candidates, who will appear better-read than perhaps they really are!

Blood transfusion for MRCPath candidates

This is not the most readable subject at the best of times and it takes a fairly revolutionary textbook to set the pulse racing when it comes to this topic. Sadly, the market is fairly stale and there are few good books to help make blood transfusion interesting.

Mollison, PL, Engelfriet, CP and Contreras, M (1993) *Blood Transfusion in Clinical Medicine*, 9th edn. Oxford: Blackwell Science.

This is the 'bible' in transfusion terms and most MRCPath candidates are advised to read it. There are good chapters (e.g. unwanted effects of blood transfusion), but most of the text is rather dull, with few illustrations.

Napier, JAF (1995) *Handbook of Blood Transfusion Therapy*, 2nd edn. Wiley, UK.

This has grown from the small HMSO handbook published several years ago and now stands at almost 500 pages. The book is well-written and reflects current practice. Information is easy to obtain and we would recommend substituting this for Mollison.

Journals

General journals

New England Journal of Medicine *Lancet* *British Medical Journal*	These contain occasional articles relevant to haematology. There have been some excellent reviews in the *New England Journal of Medicine* over recent years
British Journal of Haematology	The official journal of the British Society for Haematology. Useful annotations which MRCPath candidates should peruse before written and oral examinations
Blood	The official journal of the American Society of Hematology. Heavy-weight and difficult to read. Useful leading articles providing state-of-the-art detail for advanced haematology trainees
Blood Reviews	Published by Churchill Livingstone every 3 months. Highly readable topical reviews. Essential for MRCPath Part 1 and 2. Less useful for MRCP
Current Opinion in Hematology, *Current Science*, Adamson JW (ed.)	Now published 2-monthly, this builds up into an excellent reference source covering all aspects of haematology. Heavy North American influence, but this is no disadvantage

Other journals of value for those studying for the MRCPath examination

Bone Marrow Transplantation
Immunology Today
Journal of Clinical Oncology
Journal of Clinical Pathology
Leukemia
Leukemia Research

Scientific aspects of haematology

Cancer Genetics and Cytogenetics
Cell
EMBO Journal
Journal of Clinical Investigation
Journal of Molecular Biology
Nature
Nature Medicine
Proceedings of the National Academy of Sciences (USA)
Science

Index